The 10 Minute Yoga Solution

IRA TRIVEDI

Second Edition first published in India in 2025
by *Clever Fox Publishing Private Limited.*

P-ISBN: 978-93-6707-215-8

E-ISBN: 978-93-6707-576-0

Clever Fox Publishing Private Limited
No 1c, Vantage Plaza, Door no 1.
First Floor, LB & MG Road,
Thiruvanmiyur, Chennai 600041.

Design by Kanika Anand

Printed and bound in India

This book is dedicated to my gurus
Swami Sivananda and Swami Vishnudevananda.
I am forever in their service.

When you practise yoga, you will only want to do what is best for your body and will stay away from things that don't serve you well.

Contents

A Note from Ira

Do you want to practise yoga but wonder how and when to go about it? A class may be inaccessible – time-consuming, expensive or too far away, and even when you do join it, you may find it unimaginable (and embarrassing) to twist your body in certain ways. In an already hectic life, you may have the desire to do yoga but it may appear like an impossible dream. Not anymore. This is where the 10-minute solution comes in.

Even 10 minutes of yoga can lead to physical, mental and, eventually, spiritual transformation. My personal yoga journey is an example of this. When I first started doing yoga, now more than a decade ago, the thought of being on a yoga mat for a full hour seemed tremendously boring. I needed high-energy activities – running, squash, tennis, gymming – anything that could get my endorphins spinning and the calories burning. But all of this changed when I started doing yoga, and I started with just 10 minutes a day. The transformation was slow and subtle, almost invisible, but I stuck to the promise I had made to myself – 10 minutes of yoga every day, no matter what. The 10 minutes steadily grew to 20, 30, 60 minutes a day, and today I have a daily practise which anchors my day and grounds me in my life. Yoga has given me everything that a back-breaking gym routine or a sweaty, tedious marathon did not. Today I am at the pinnacle of my physical fitness. I have recovered from a serious neck injury, acquired washboard abs that I had once only dreamed of (also lost hope of), and my skin, hair and other vital stats are keeping as well as I could ever wish for. And this is just on the physical level.

I am a much more peaceful and content person than I ever was before. As I learnt to control my body and breath through yoga, I also learnt how to steady my mind. And when I learnt to steady my mind, I learnt how to control my anger, my fear, my selfish and vain desires. Yoga has put me on a trajectory of self-discovery, a path on which I have found balance, joy and myself. And it all started with just 10 minutes a day.

What can 10 minutes of yoga do?

Even a short 10-minute practise can yield tremendous results. It can lead to weight loss, it can lead to chiselled abs, it can remedy back pain and help with chronic diseases like diabetes or high blood pressure, it can improve your eyesight and it can even help you cope with heartbreak. More than anything else, it can help you lead a better, more balanced life. Like many alternative forms of wellness, yoga steadily lets you

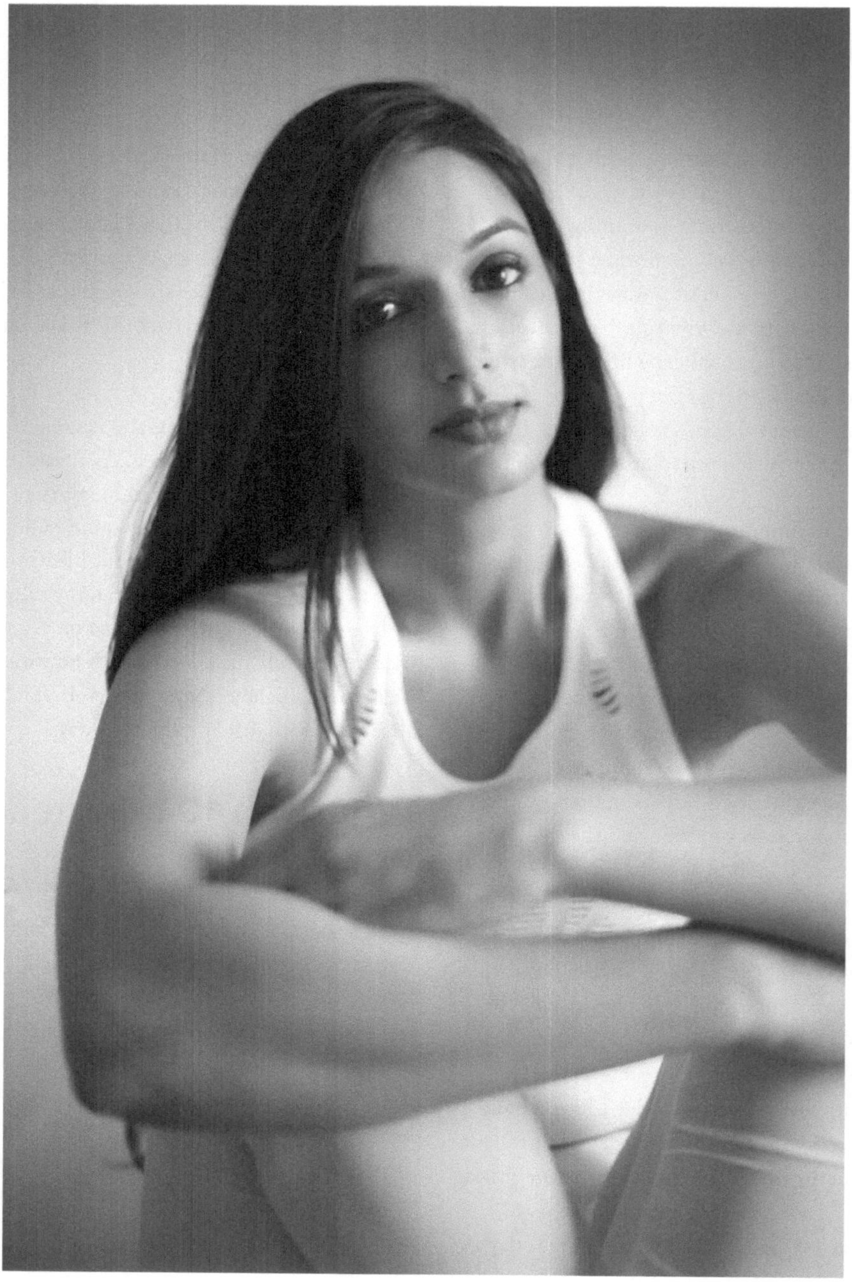

progress on your path of self-improvement and creates permanent positive change with no nasty side effects.

This book is designed to do a few things.

INTRODUCE YOU TO YOGA BASICS

What is an asana? Pranayama? How is yoga different from going to the gym? What is all the hype about? This book will answer all these questions and help you kick-start your yoga practise by offering an effective personalized yoga solution that can be carried out in the comfort and convenience of your own home.

WORK ON SPECIFIC AILMENTS

Whatever your problem is, yoga can help cure it. This book presents to you twenty-five yoga cures for twenty-five of the most common lifestyle issues of our time. Whether your problem is physical, mental or emotional, yoga can cure, help and prevent.

GET YOU STARTED ON YOUR YOGA JOURNEY

This book has simplified elements of ancient yoga practises to make them as user-friendly and time effective as possible. Begin with just 10 minutes a day, and gradually increase the intensity and level of your practise to a comfortable pace that is perfectly tailored to your lifestyle. Like a salad, mix and match, and toss what is irrelevant at your discretion. As you start practising, you will learn what your body needs and understand how to work on it.

And most importantly...

THIS BOOK TAKES YOU AN INCH FORWARD ON THE SPIRITUAL JOURNEY THAT IS LIFE

Is yoga a spiritual practise? Yes, it is. Physical purification is perhaps the easiest and surest path towards mental and emotional purification. When you breathe correctly, you reduce stress levels; when you balance on your toes, you balance your mind; when you challenge yourself by trying a difficult asana, you face your fears.

Yoga prepares and disciplines your body and mind for a deeper spiritual experience. Through the purging of negative thoughts and habits, you begin to declutter your mind and thus your life.

Whatever your personal goals are, I guarantee that they can be achieved through yoga – whether it's weight loss, increasing flexibility in your body, building strength or tone. Even something like hair growth and skin problems can be improved through the practise of yoga. However, yoga is not a temporary or instant quick fix. Instead, it is a sustainable practise that works internally to bring about permanent change. With a little time (only 10 minutes) and a dash of patience, yoga will yield benefits that can, and will, last a lifetime.

The Yoga Life

I was overweight, I had bad skin and was losing hair. None of my clothes fit me and my constant state of agitation was ruining my personal relationships. I had just moved back to India from the US and I was depressed, lethargic and had a major case of writer's block. Overall, my life was utterly imbalanced. This was my state of being when I first began my yoga practise.

Ten years later, I am at my ideal weight. I eat healthier and never fight to ward off cravings. It may sound bizarre but I only crave what is good for my body and my hair and my skin are not just under control, but fabulous. I have a healthy attitude towards my work – I work hard but am detached from the outcome of the results – and often I find myself floating on a creative high. I have better control over my emotions and have realized that there is nothing in this world, or in this life, that should make me unhappy. No matter how clichéd it sounds, I've also realized that no matter what the circumstances, or how dreary the situation, life can truly be a joy every step of the way.

A simple yoga and meditation practise helped trigger my transformation. My time spent at the Sivananda Ashram taught me that yoga is not just a physical practise but a lifestyle, and that it is crucial to inculcate yoga into all aspects of your life. This may sound daunting (you may wonder why you even picked up this book, it is the *10-Minute Yoga Solution* after all) but it is much easier – and less time consuming – than it sounds. The yogic life happens organically and naturally. And it begins with just 10 minutes a day.

Perhaps the simplest way to explain it all is through the five points of yoga.

Yoga means union. That is the meaning of the word. A union of body, mind, soul, a union with our soul, a union with Brahman – the supreme soul.

The five essential points of yoga are:

1. proper breath
2. proper relaxation
3. proper diet
4. proper exercise
5. positive thinking

These points are interlinked. Each one leads to the other, and practise of yoga helps nurture all five. While physically practising yoga, you always focus on your breath. As you hold the asana, you learn how to relax deeply. Asanas work on your internal organs and hormone systems, which in turn helps control sugar cravings and unhealthy eating habits. Asana practise, even a short one, leads you away from negative feelings of anger, anxiety and fear towards positivity and joy. A good diet will come naturally. When you practise yoga, you will only want to do what is best for your body and will stay away from things that don't serve you well.

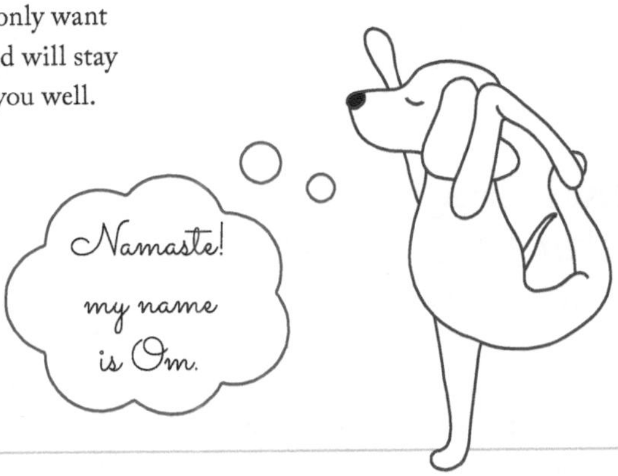

Yoga is not about touching your toes, its about what you learn on the way down.

What Is an Asana?

Patanjali, author of the popular text *Yoga Sutras*, said, '*Sthira, sukham asanam*,' an asana should always be steady and comfortable. It must always be done with mental awareness and by coordinating your breath. The longer you hold the asana the more effective it will be. Yoga is about cultivating stillness in motion. The meditative nature of yoga is also what sets it apart from other physical practices where you are focused on the external rather than on the internal.

Why is yoga better than going to the gym?

Yoga not only works on the outside to give you a perfectly toned body, but it also works on your inside – on your circulatory system, on your respiratory system, on your hormonal systems, on your digestive system to synchronize your bodily functions. It also works on reducing stress through breath and relaxation. At a subtler, more subconscious level, yoga also works on your prana, the vital life force purifying your body and mind.

Asanas have healing properties. The benefits are endless, but the ones I consider most important are listed here.

PHYSICAL BENEFITS

1. When you do inverted postures you kick-start circulation. This not only prevents ailments such as obesity, peripheral vascular disease and high blood cholesterol, but also rejuvenates and revitalizes your systems.
2. Chest-expanding asanas help you breathe correctly and release tension.
3. Twisting postures massage the internal organs of your body.
4. Asanas work on muscles to free them of lactic acid and release tension.
5. Asanas work on lymphatic systems to detoxify your body.
6. Per Ayurveda, the stomach is where all diseases begin and end, so doing regular yoga helps in keeping your digestive system strong.
7. Asanas work on balancing the hormonal systems leading to better skin, hair and regular menstrual cycles.

EMOTIONAL BENEFITS

1. Hormonal balance leads to more balanced moods.
2. Certain asanas work on the pancreas, stabilizing blood sugar levels.

3 Asanas stimulate the release of happy hormones like serotonin or endorphins, hormones which make us feel good.

SUBCONSCIOUS BENEFITS

1 Mental control instils discipline

2 Focus

3 Concentration

4 Creative high (this book is hopefully a testament to this!)

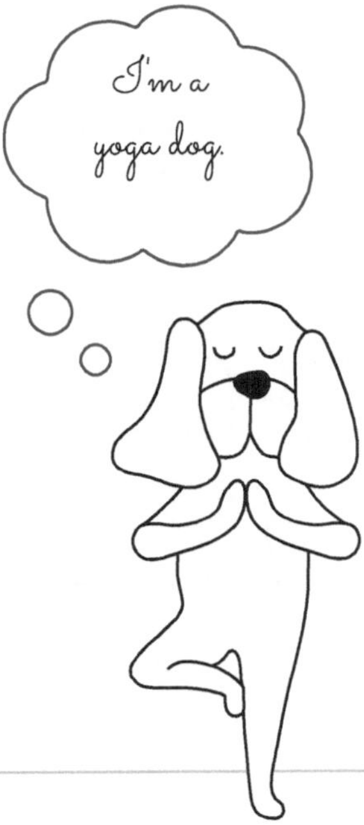

SOME TIPS FOR YOUR ASANA PRACTISE AS YOU EMBARK ON YOUR YOGA JOURNEY.

1. Push yourself, but never too much. You should always be steady and mindful in your asana practise. Like relationships, yoga positions require work but they should never be forced.

2. Yoga cannot, and will not lead, to injuries if you are self-aware.

3. Always use your breath. This is important. Without synchronizing your breath, movement in yoga and asana practise is not as beneficial.

4. Yoga is not gymnastics. It involves slow, balanced movements that focus on the steady rhythm of the body with the breath.

5. Yoga is not about achieving complex asanas. It is far more beneficial to gain mastery over the simple ones as a solid foundation to a healthy yoga practise.

6. Relaxation is a critical part of yoga. Make sure you do Shavasana frequently.

How to Use this Book

1. Begin with the 10-minute solution given for the specific ailment you hope to prevent or cure.

2. With gradual practise you may feel that you need more time, especially with the breathing and pranayama practises. Remember, this book is meant to get you kick-started with your yoga journey, but hopefully that is not where it will end.

3. Try growing your practise from 10 minutes to 15 minutes, then from 20 minutes to 30 minutes and onwards. This will happen organically and from within. You will not have to push yourself too much.

4. If you don't have even 10 minutes, then take an asana or two out of the book and incorporate them in your routine. Some yoga is better than no yoga.

5. The goal of this book is to introduce you to yoga and its umpteen benefits. A daily 10-minute practise will put you on the path of cure and prevention, but remember, yoga, like anything good, takes times and works from the inside out for deep-lasting benefits. So, stick with your practise and if you're ever feeling demotivated drop me an email, Tweet or Facebook message and I will always be happy to chat with you.

MY YOGA PRACTICE.

I practise twelve asanas every day. I have been following the same yoga routine for the past decade and I intend to practise these for the next ten years, and the ten after that. Basically, however long my body will allow me to practise. While yoga keeps me fit, toned and healthy, I now do my practise because of how it makes me feel versus how it makes me look. The changes that have taken place in my body, mind and inner-self have been subtle yet profound, and I can now say with great confidence that yoga has changed my life. It has made me a better person; it has made me a better writer and it has brought me closer to discovering and realizing my purpose on planet earth.

Here and now is where yoga begins.

Prana: May the Force Be with You

What is pranayama? Why this emphasis on breathing? Don't we all just breathe anyway? Prana is the vital or life force, the *chi*. Prana is the life-giving energy; it is that which keeps you alive. *Pra* means constant and *An* means movement, so *prana* means constant motion. *Yama* translates to control; hence with the practise of pranayama you essentially learn how to control and channel this vital energy using your breath.

While we all breathe, how we breathe is not something we normally think about. But it can have a huge impact on your energy level, on your mood and on your overall health. Cities are getting increasingly polluted and it is important now more than ever to pay attention to your breath. Try some of the simple exercises in this book and you will begin to witness a shift in your life and health by focusing on the simplest of things – your breath.

The reality is that most of us do not breathe correctly. We breathe shallow breaths, taking in only a small portion of the oxygen that your lungs are capable of, and of what you need. This leads to fatigue, lethargy, bad moods and, eventually, health problems. For years, I didn't breathe correctly. I suffered from major sinus issues and no matter how many pills I took, I couldn't fix my problems. Once I started doing yoga and pranayama, all my sinus issues disappeared. I always begin my day with a practise of pranayama and I have discovered, my own life being the example – that 5 minutes of pranayama a day, keeps the doctor away.

Doing pranayama may be a bit of an alien concept to you. It used to be for me. I wondered how breathing exercises could benefit me and if it was anything more than some yoga marketing gimmick. Over time I discovered that pranayama not only helped me build lung strength (I was a runner back then, so this was important) and keep respiratory diseases at bay, but that it also led to weight loss, curbed unhealthy cravings and made me mentally strong. Most importantly, pranayama felt deeply meditative and helped build my daily meditation practise.

Be yoga.

In the beginning, you may think pranayama is slow and boring, but the benefits of this are deeply transforming, even more so than the asana practise. Over time, ten years to be precise, I have realized that a pranayama practise is as important if not more important than asana practise itself. If I have only 5 minutes to set aside for yoga, then I will choose pranayama over asana any day. And there are visible physical benefits as well. For example, Kapalabhati, a cleansing kriya that you will see frequently in this book, is also excellent for toning the abs. Fifty pumps through the Kapalabhati kriya is equivalent to the same amount of sit ups. And you don't even have to break out in a sweat!

Deep breaths are like little love notes to your body.

In this book, I outline basic pranayama or kriyas (warm-up exercises) and suggest you do them for short durations of time, typically 1-3 minutes. But the more pranayama you do, the better. And if there is one part of your practise that you can give more time to, the pranayama portion of the routine is what you should increase.

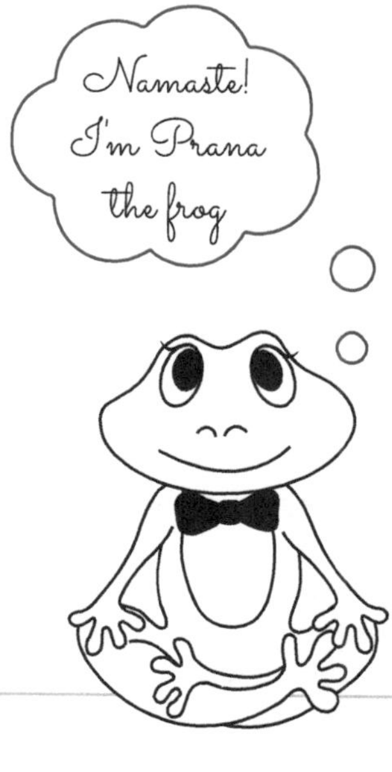

A MESSAGE FROM PRANA THE FROG

The prana is a vital force in your life. It is so important that the *Bhagavad Gita* dedicates an entire section to this, and there is an entire Upanishad focused on this as well!

The Wobbly Mind

The *Bhagavad Gita* describes meditation as the easiest and quickest way to reach the divine, and while the focus is not on meditation per se in this book, practising yoga can be a form of meditation.

For many ancient gurus, the main goal of doing asanas was to increase their flexibility so they could sit in meditation for long hours without any physical discomfort. Pranayama was aimed at preparing the mind before meditation, and certain pranayama introduced in the book were used to generate heat in the body and rid it of hunger so yogis could sit for long uninterrupted hours in their quest for self-realization.

My students often tell me that meditation is impossible for them, that when they try to sit still, they are immediately assaulted by a million thoughts and ideas, and when they get up, they are often more disturbed than when they sat down because of the million new thoughts that the million old thoughts generated. For all of you who suffer from the wobbly mind syndrome (though I have had a decade-long yoga practise, there are still days when my mind won't sit still at all), a yoga practise can be a great way to experience meditation. I believe that a yoga practise lays a good foundation for the body not just by building spinal strength and flexibility but by balancing a wobbly mind. For example, when you strike a balancing posture such as Tadasana or the Tree Pose you use your breath to focus your mind. You are then subconsciously balancing and calming a wobbly mind. Yoga helps strengthen the mind, preparing you slowly (and surely) for the day when you are ready to sit down and meditate.

A yoga practise also helps the mind become mindful. There are so many distractions these days. Phones, social media, email, TV – the electronic world is constantly screaming out for attention and the power of concentration is at an all-time low. For the 10 minutes that you get on the mat, try to be in the here and the now. Try to focus on your breath and your body. You will be amazed at how far practising just 10 minutes of mindfulness will take you. Yoga can help develop mindfulness and keep you connected to your inner self in a world that is becoming increasingly outwardly connected.

No matter what my state of mind, my yoga practise has never once failed me. Just ten minutes of yoga, and I leave the world behind, entering a calm, beautiful, peaceful place that I can carry with me wherever I go. This is where I want to take you too.

yoga for beginners

Have you always wanted to do yoga, but been scared off by the twisting, bending and strange contortions? Petrified to enter a class and get left behind? Or worse – make a total fool of yourself? Worry no more! This 10-minute yoga solution is designed for those of you who don't know the Y of yoga but wish to get down on the mat.

These may look like simple asanas but they are super-effective with deep physical and mental benefits. So, begin your yoga journey with this simple routine and allow yoga to transform your life.

As you begin to feel more confident, you can increase the time that you spend on each of these practises. This guide will allow you to adjust the intensity of your practise at your own pace, growing as fast as you can, and as slowly as you need.

your notes:

01 – TWO MINUTES

belly breath

instructions

1. Sit up straight in a comfortable, relaxed posture
2. Place the right hand gently on the stomach. Resting the left hand on the knee bring together the thumb and forefinger in Gyan mudra
3. Inhale deeply allowing the stomach to expand slowly like a balloon. Release and exhale, allowing the air to move up the chest, throat and out the nose

Continue breathing mindfully this way for two minutes, focusing on the rhythm of your breath and the steady expansion and contraction of your abdomen.

benefits

1. Increased oxygenation
2. Deep and sound relaxation

contraindications: None

I am always shocked by the number of people in my classes who breathe incorrectly. They breathe in from their chests rather than their diaphragms. Chest breathing is shallow and allows for a very small percentage of oxygen to be taken into your bodies. Belly breath is a beneficial and therapeutic exercise which teaches you to inhale and exhale correctly. A small change in your breathing habits can make a significant difference in your life by increasing the efficiency with which your body uses oxygen for basic daily functions.

Diaphragmatic breathing is the most natural way of breathing. Observe how a very young baby breathes – they will use their diaphragm and belly with each breath. Relearning to use your diaphragm during breathing and to reduce your rate of breathing is an important first step in managing the symptoms of anxiety, anger and panic.

In my yoga classes, only one out of seven beginner students know how to breathe correctly! Years of stress, anxiety, tension and fear constrict your breathing till you breathe only from your chest. This limits your oxygen intake and affects the optimal potential of your health.

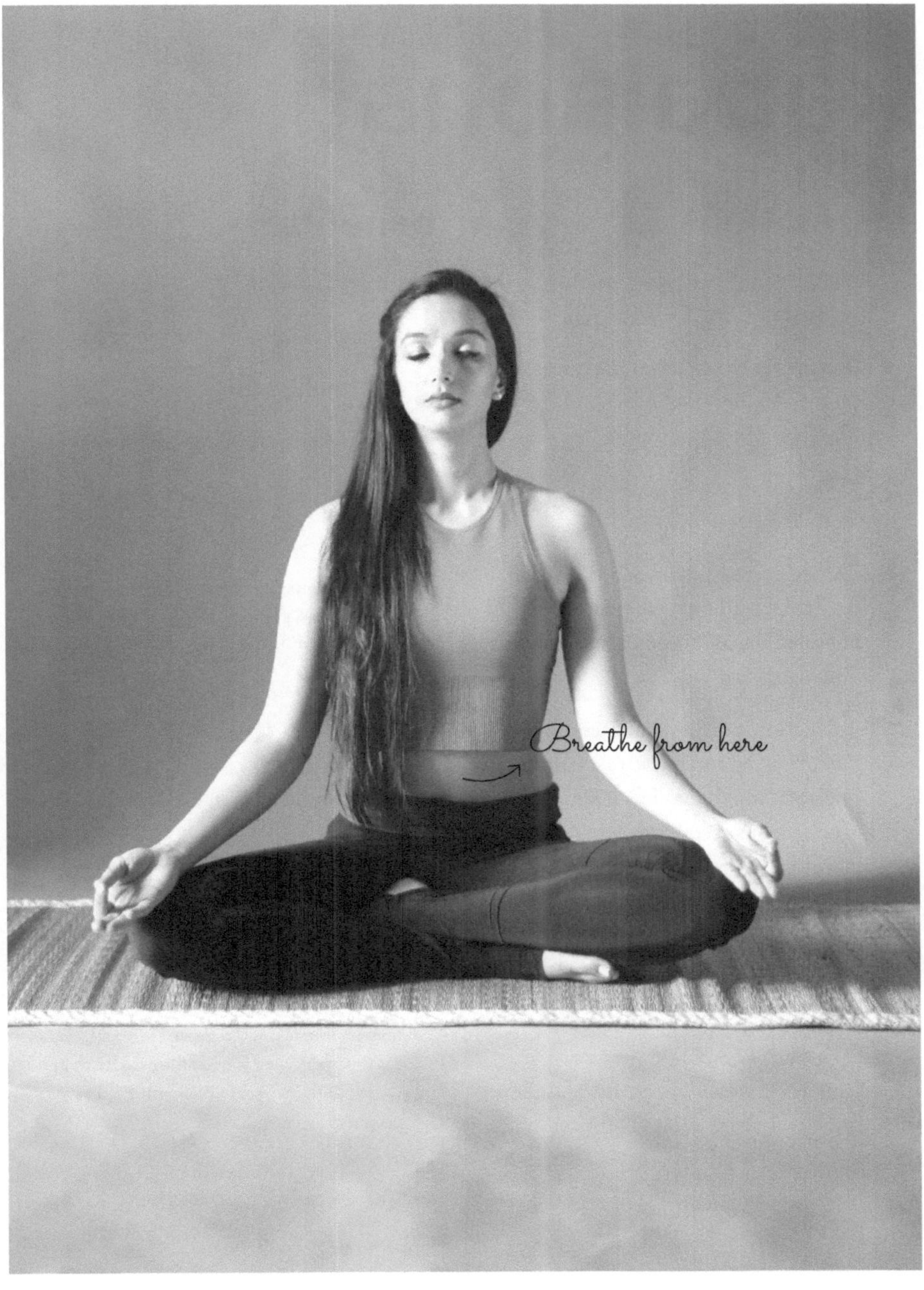
Breathe from here

02 – TWO MINUTES

kapalabhati

instructions

1. Sit up straight in a comfortable, relaxed posture
2. Resting both hands on the knees, bring together the thumb and forefinger in Gyan mudra
3. Close the eyes and take a few deep breaths
4. Inhale deeply (only when you begin) and contracting the abdominal muscles, exhale through both nostrils, forcing the air out
5. Inhalation should take place *passively* by automatic relaxation of the abdominal muscles. It should be spontaneous recoil, involving no active effort
6. After completing 20 rapid breaths stop and resume normal breathing pace. This is one complete round

You can gradually build up your practise by increasing the number of rounds, and the breaths taken in each round. Move from 20 breaths initially to 30 breaths and so forth.

benefits

1. Improves blood circulation
2. Increases oxygenation
3. Strengthens the lungs
4. Stimulates the digestive organs
5. Tones the abdominal muscles

contraindications: Respiratory disorders, circulatory disorders, hernias, gastric ulcers. This kriya is not recommended during the first 3 months of pregnancy

This kriya is a fantastic way of getting that 'yoga-glow'. In Sanskrit, Kapalabhati means shining skull. Doing this on a regular basis should become an essential part of your beauty routine.

YOGA TIP:

Note that Kapalabhati is an almost involuntary response, with the abdominal muscles mimicking a pumping action. If you get this right, then you get the practise right. Often, this is the part of the practise that people struggle with the most.

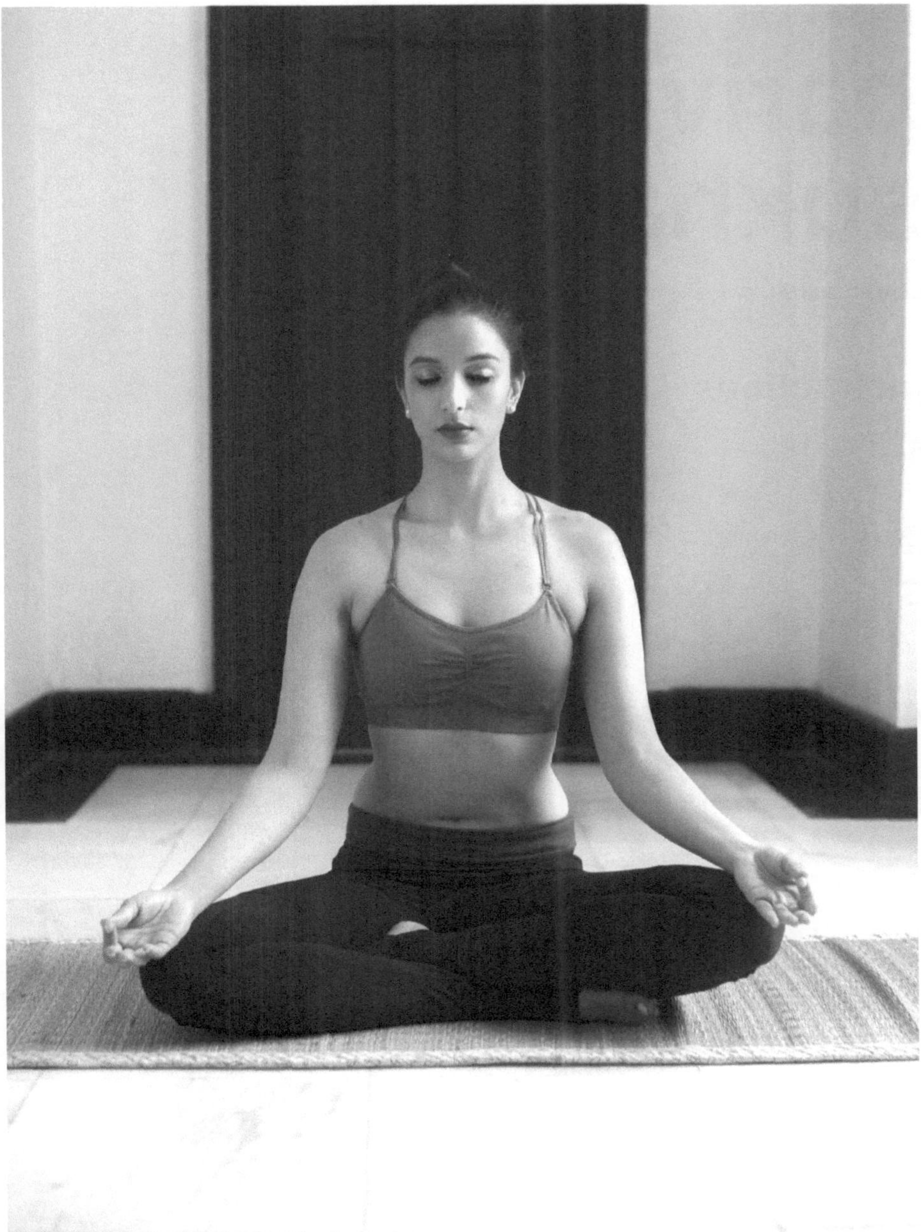

03 – ONE MINUTE

parivrtta sukhasana

SEATED SPINAL TWIST

instructions

1. Sit in sukhasana or a simple crossed leg position
2. Inhale and raise the left arm
3. Exhale, place the left hand on the right knee, and the right hand on the hip for support
4. Inhale and return to centre facing forward
5. Repeat on the other side

benefits

1. Increases flexibility in the back and spine
2. Relieves tension in the neck, shoulders and back
3. Stretches the chest
4. Massages the internal organs stimulating detox

contraindications: Severe neck or back injuries

your notes:

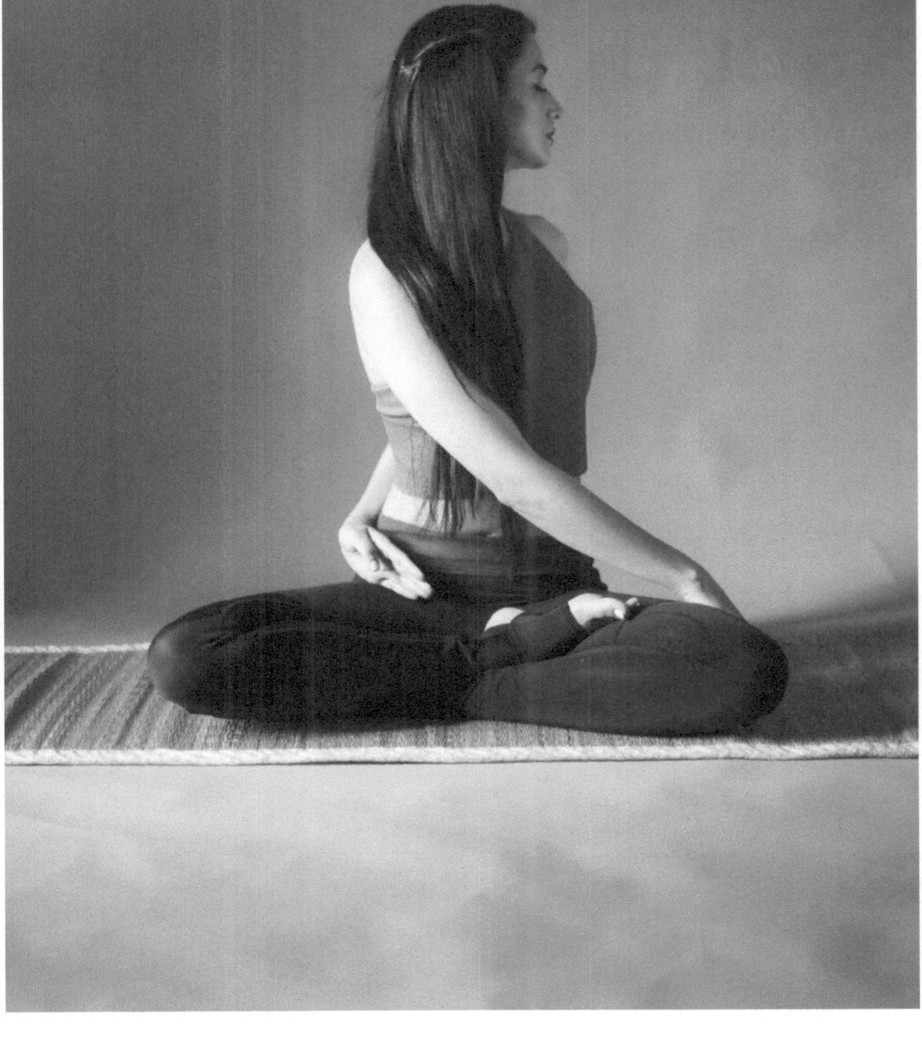

04 – ONE MINUTE

supta padangustha asana

HAMSTRING STRETCH WITH THE BELT

instructions

1. Lying on the back, raise the left leg and place the centre of a belt or towel around the arch of the left foot
2. Keeping the right leg on the floor, raise the left leg toward the ceiling, as high as you comfortably can
3. Hold for 5 breaths
4. Repeat on the other side

benefits

1. Strengthens and tones the hamstrings and calves

contraindications: Knee injuries, ligament injuries (leg)

your notes:

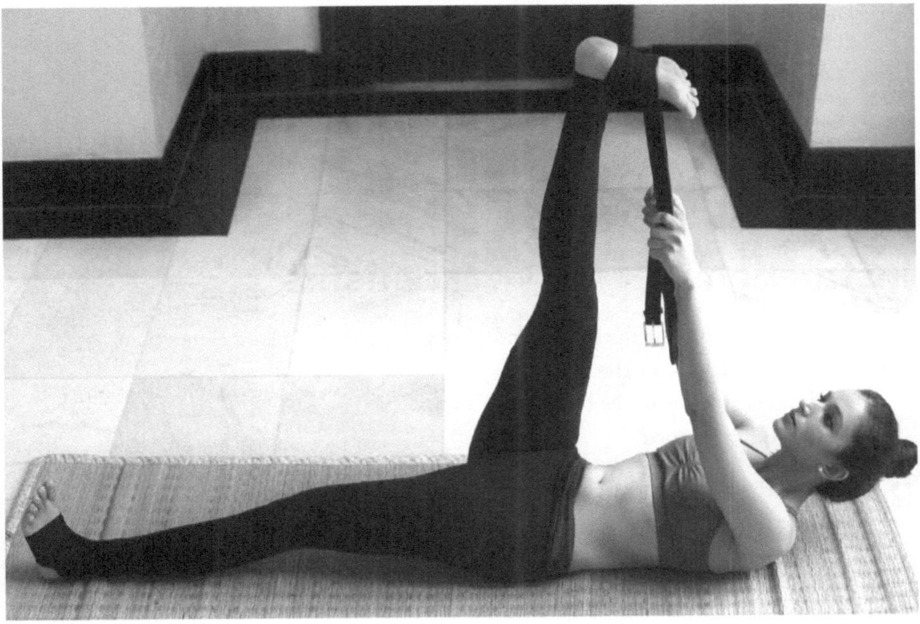

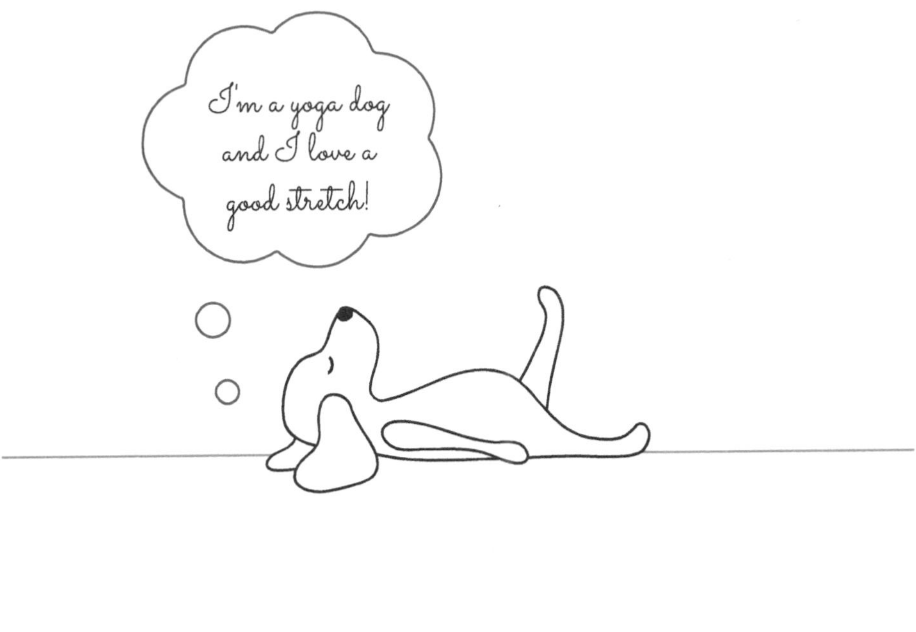
I'm a yoga dog
and I love a
good stretch!

05 – ONE MINUTE

sarvangasana

SHOULDER STAND

instructions

1. Lie flat on the back with the legs and feet together and place the arms and hands on either side of the body with the palms facing down
2. Raise both legs and move the legs over the head
3. Push down on the arms, raising the hips up and taking the legs further back
4. In the final position, the weight of the body rests on the shoulders, neck and elbows
5. Gaze up towards the toes
6. Stay here and breathe

benefits

1. Improves blood circulation
2. Regulates the thyroid function
3. Corrects imbalances in the nervous system
4. Improves posture

contraindications: High blood pressure, circulatory diseases, inflammation of the eye, spinal injuries, vertigo, pregnancy

YOGA TIP:
If you find this asana challenging, begin by doing the Viparita Karani (page 200) and then gradually build up to this asana.

YOGA FACT:
Inversions have *huge* benefits as they reverse the ageing effect of gravity on your body. So, make sure you don't skip this one.

your notes:

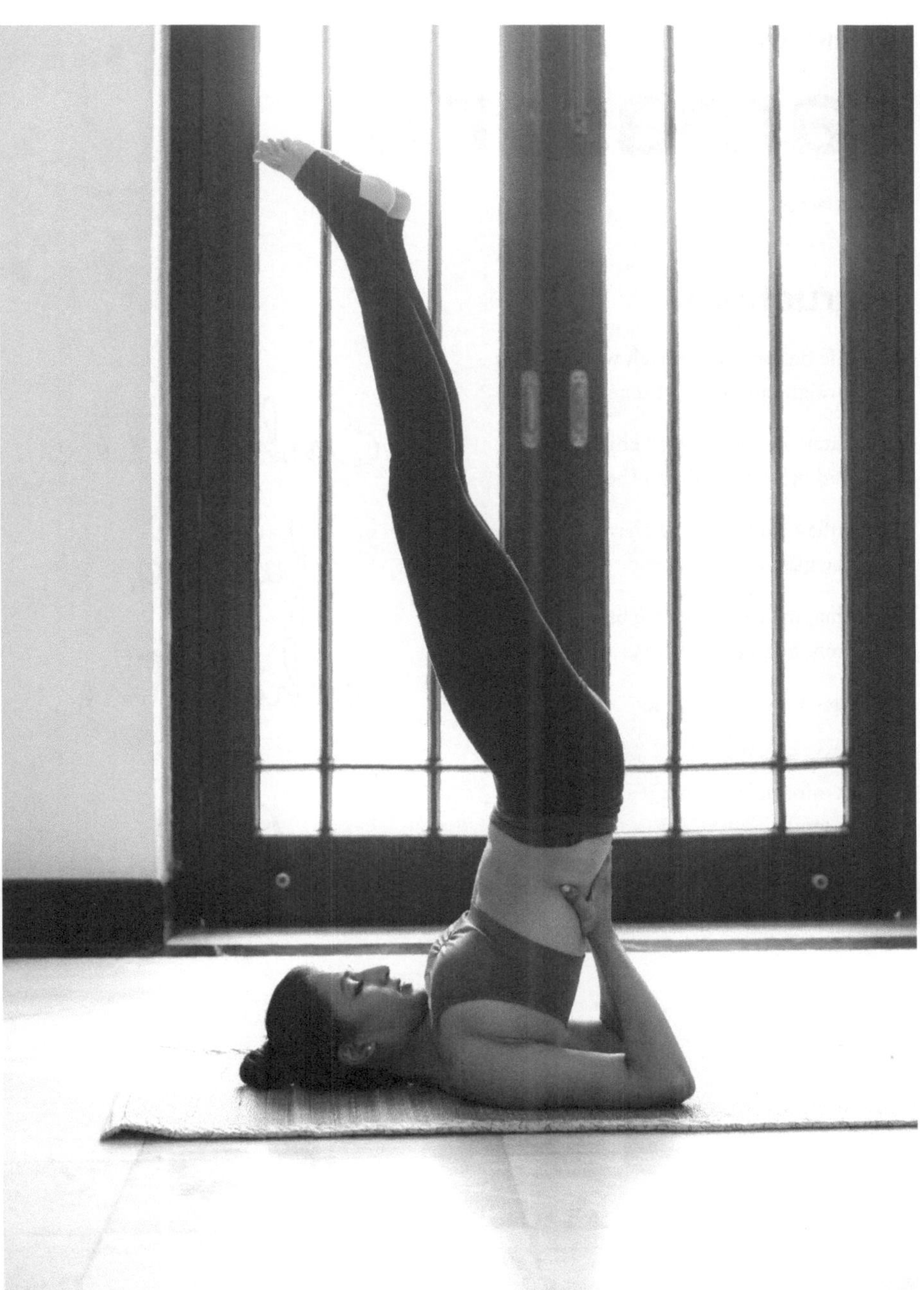

06 – ONE MINUTE

sarpasana

SNAKE POSE

instructions

1 Lie flat on the stomach with the legs straight and the feet together

2 Interlace the fingers behind the back and place the chin on the ground

3 Inhale and raise the chest, keeping the gaze straight ahead

4 Imagine the hands are being pulled from behind

5 Stay here and breathe

6 Hold this for as long as you are comfortable, even if it's for just a few seconds

7 Come down, take a few breaths and come up again

Inhale the future, exhale the past.

your notes:

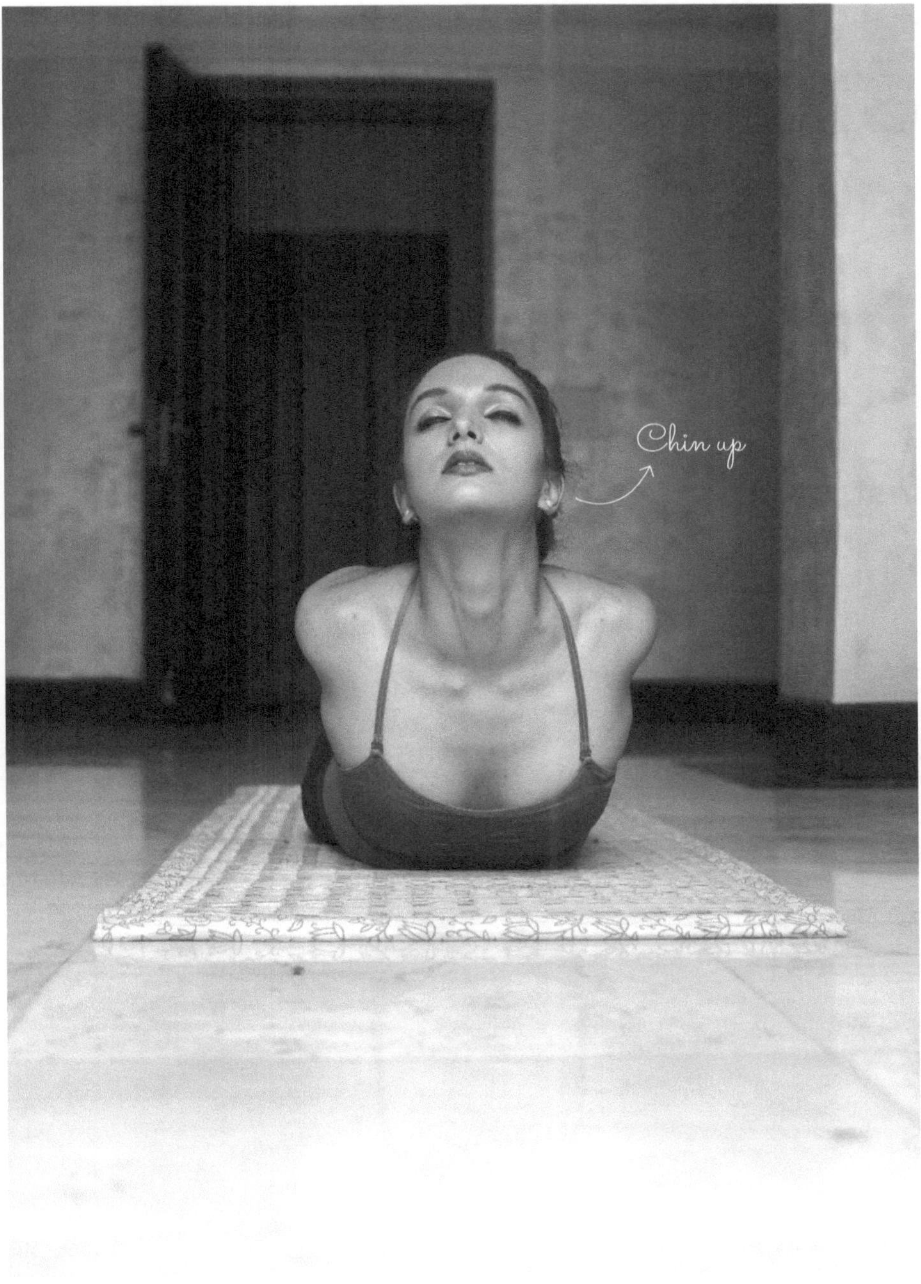
Chin up

07 – ONE MINUTE

ardha uttana asana

TABLE TOP POSE

instructions

1 Standing with the feet together, inhale and raise the arms above the head

2 Exhale and bend at the waist, extending the arms straight out

3 The body should form a 90-degree angle

4 Stay here and breathe

benefits

1 Stretches the leg muscles

2 Improves flexibility in the spine

3 Improves balance

contraindications: Spinal injuries

The Table Top Pose saved my spine. At twenty-five, I was saddled with a spinal problem so severe that I had to wear a neck brace for 3 months. I started with this asana to regain my spinal health. I performed it against any table that I could find, resting my palms on the table so I could go deeper into the stretch.

your notes:

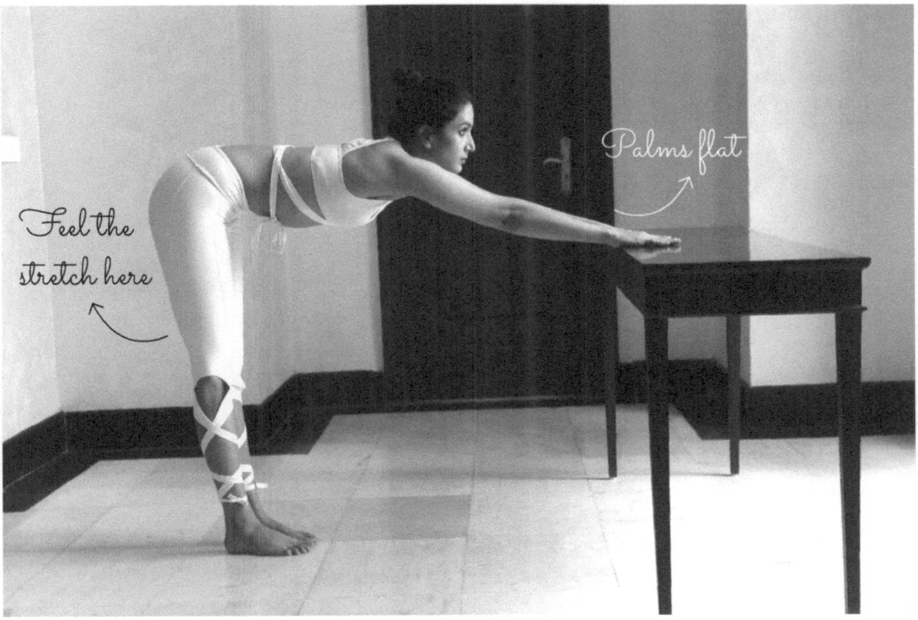

The journey towards yoga and spiritual growth begins with just one asana a day

08 – ONE MINUTE

shavasana

CORPSE POSE

instructions

1 Lie flat on the back with arms relaxed on either side of the body, palms facing upward

2 The legs should be sprawled outward and the feet apart

3 The head and neck should be aligned

4 Inhale and exhale and relax the entire body

5 To further deepen the relaxation, actively contract and relax different parts of the body

6 Contract the muscles in the feet, and relax. Contract the calves and thighs, and relax. Contract the pelvic muscles, the buttocks and relax. Clench the fists, contract the arms, and relax. Contract, contract, contract, and relax. Contract the back, the neck, the shoulders, and relax. Lift the head off the ground, and relax. Contract, contract, contract, and relax. Contract the muscles in the face, and relax. Contract the entire body. Contract, contract, contract and relax. Recite this mentally

7 Inhale and exhale deeply, counting backwards from 10 gradually down to 1

benefits

1 Calms the mind and helps alleviate stress and depression

2 Relaxes the body

3 Alleviates headaches, fatigue, and insomnia

4 Reduces blood pressure

contraindications: Back injury (bend the knees as in the Butterfly Pose to ease any pressure on the spine). Pregnancy (raise the head and chest with a pillow or bolster to provide support in this pose)

your notes:

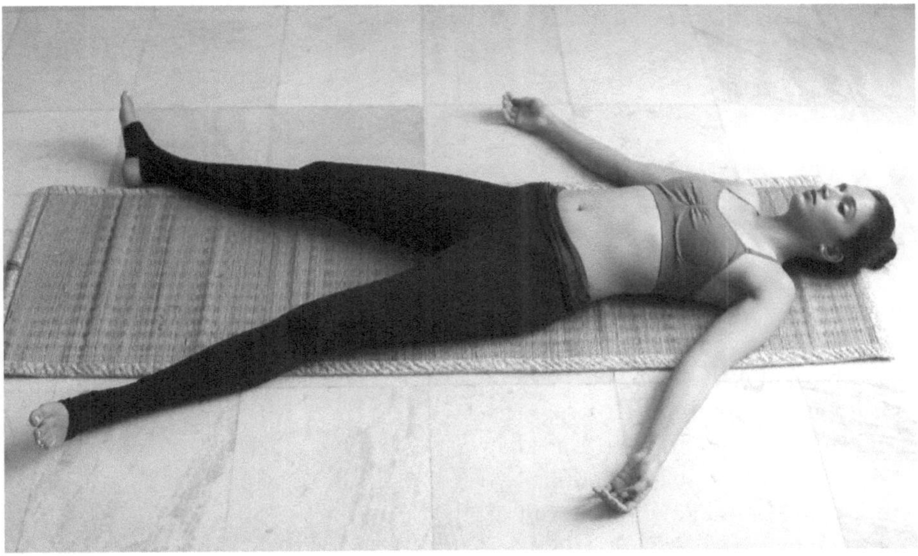

There is no correct ratio for how far apart the arms and legs should be in Shavasana. Use the picture as a reference and adjust accordingly. Do note, however, that spreading the limbs too far apart creates pressure on the spine.

Though the Corpse Pose or Shavasana looks very simple, it is considered by many yogis to be the most difficult asana of them all. You are meant to be as still as a corpse (Shava means corpse in Sanskrit) and to achieve this can be a major challenge! But keep at it and you shall persevere...

Stillness is the ruler of movement. – Lao Tzu

hair yoga

Yoga is truly a wonder drug. Not only can it get you fit and healthy, a practise helps stabilize your hormones, preventing hair loss, thinning and even greying. Certain yoga asanas promote circulation, stimulating blood flow to the scalp and thereby increases hair growth. Relaxation through yoga asanas can help eradicate the multitude of hair problems that come with stress. Beat all your hair problems with this simple 10-minute yoga solution.

your notes:

01 – TWO MINUTES

shashank asana

HARE POSE

instructions

1. Begin in Vajrasana (Diamond Pose)
2. Spread the knees apart so that the toes of both feet are touching
3. Inhale and raise the arms over the head
4. Exhale bringing the forehead to the ground. Extend the arms out on either side of the head
5. Stay here and breathe

benefits

1. Improves blood circulation
2. Relaxes the pelvis and improves reproductive health
3. Aids in digestion and relieves constipation

contraindications: Spinal disc herniation, vertigo, high blood pressure, circulatory diseases

your notes:

YOGA FACT:
There is a reason why hares are such soft, furry creatures; they do this asana all the time.

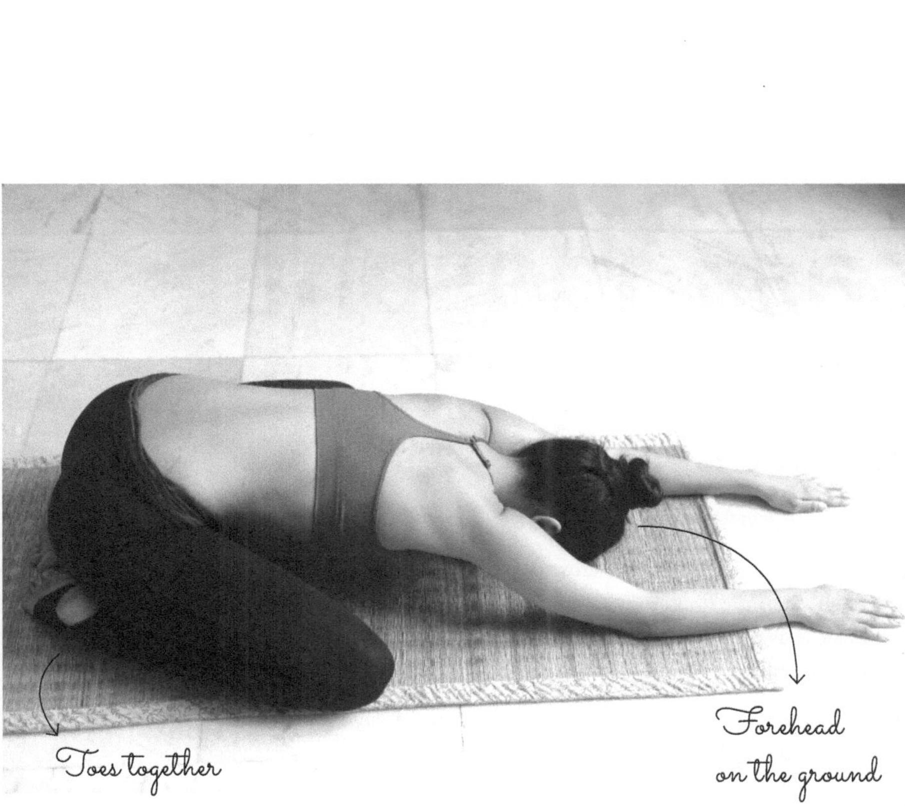

If you are losing balance in a yoga pose reach higher. It will steady you. This is true not just in your practice but also in your life.

02 – TWO MINUTES

sasangasana

RABBIT POSE

instructions

1 Begin in Vajrasana (Diamond Pose)

2 Bend forward bringing the crown of the head to the floor, moving inward as close as possible to the knees as the hips are raised up

3 Extend the arms on either side of the body and hold the ankles

4 Stay here and breathe

benefits

1 Regulates hormonal imbalance

2 Improves blood circulation

contraindications: Neck injuries, knee injuries

your notes:

If you don't bend, you break.

your notes:

*Yoga is like life.
It is balance of holding
on and letting go.*

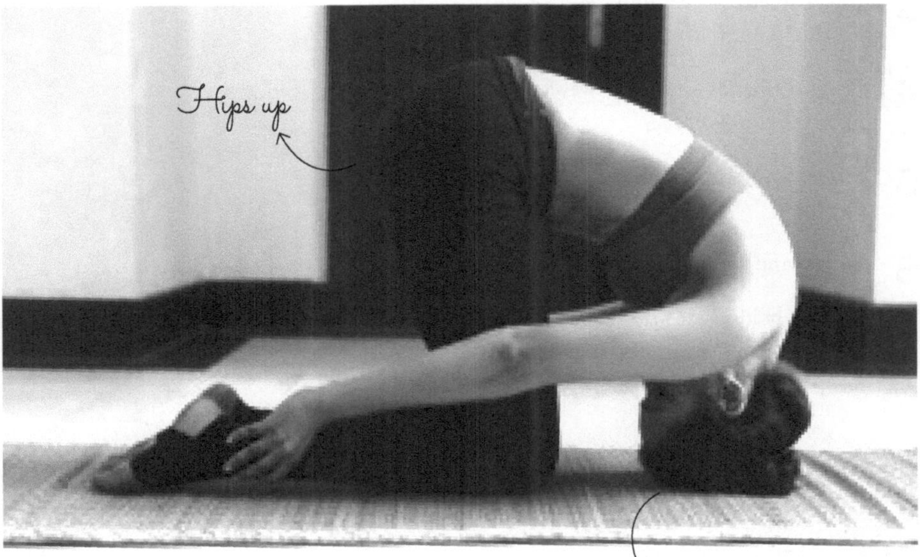

03 – TWO MINUTES

sethu bandhasana

BRIDGE POSE

instructions

1. Lying on the back, bend both knees and place the feet flat on the floor, hip width apart
2. Bring the arms alongside the body with the palms facing downwards
3. Inhale, press the feet into the floor and lift the hips up
4. Bring the hands onto the lower back for support if you wish
5. Stay here for 10 seconds continuing to breathe
6. Exhale and come down
7. Start by holding this asana for 10 seconds. Come down, rest for a few breaths and then come back again

benefits

1. Regulates hormonal imbalance
2. Stretches the lower back

contraindications: Neck injuries, back injuries, knee injuries

your notes:

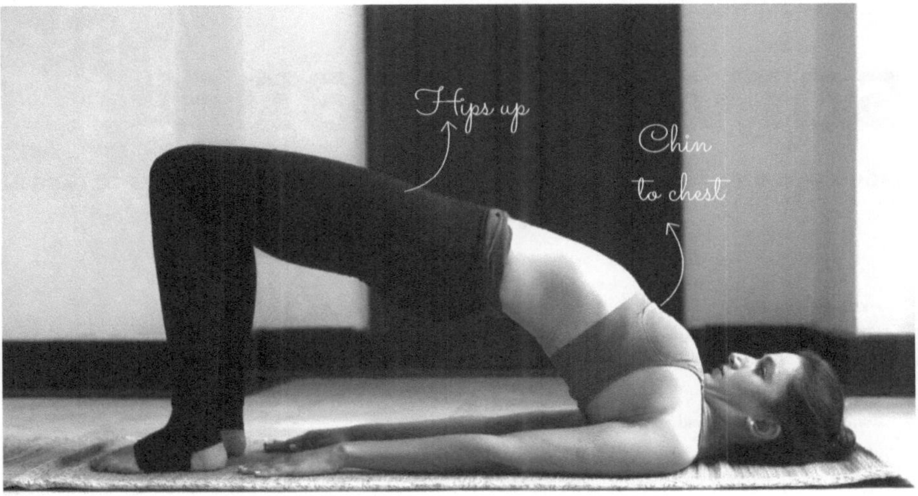

Yoga is not a workout,
it is a work in.

your notes:

04 – TWO MINUTES

sarvangasana

SHOULDER STAND

REFER TO PAGE 22

YOGA FACT:
The Sarvangasana is known as the mother of all asanas because of its multiple benefits. The main benefit of this asana is that it works wonders on your thyroid gland.

your notes:

05 – TWO MINUTES

mudra: bal vyayam yoga

The *Bal Vyayam* is the simplest yoga technique for hair growth. All you need to do is to rub the fingernails of both hands together and you will stimulate hair growth.

In ancient texts, this hand posture is known as the *Prasanna mudra*. When you rub finger nails together, you stimulate energy points in your body, which leads to better hair growth.

instructions

1. Curl the fingers inwards so that the fingers point towards the palm
2. Bring the hands together so that the nails of all the fingers touch each other
3. Rub vigorously and with focus for 2 minutes

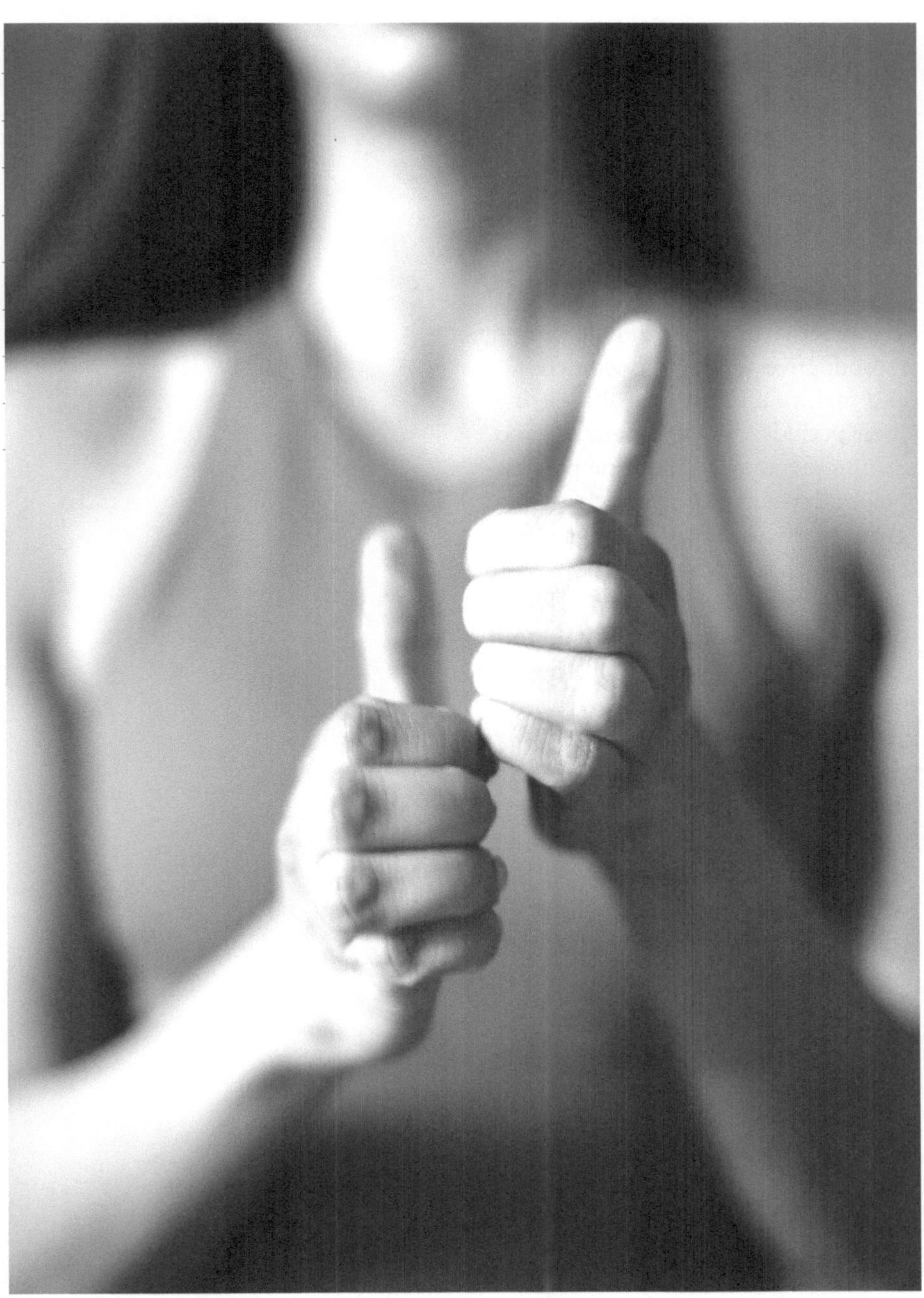

yoga for women

The practise of yoga can help promote reproductive wellness in women and maintain optimal health during their periods, during pregnancy and during menopause. Routine practise helps alleviates symptoms that are associated with fertility cycles – so much so that teachers specializing in prenatal yoga are trained to ease the period of pregnancy that is vital to the growth and development of a healthy baby. Personally, it was yoga which gave me the body that I wanted – not the hundred other things I tried. I find that yoga suits women's bodies, it helps tone but prevents bulking up. It also helps get rid of pesky blotting, which can give the appearance of weight. Below are five essential asanas that every woman should incorporate into her daily routine.

your notes:

YOGA FOR PMS

A monthly ordeal you are all too familiar with, PMS (Premenstrual Syndrome) can cause a whole range of symptoms from physical discomfort to emotional mood swings. Just a few minutes of yoga a day can help mitigate the effect of these symptoms on the body and eliminate the need for any form of medication. I, like so many women that I know, suffered from the worst period cramps and PMS pain. A regular yoga practise has helped bring my menstrual rhythm under control.

01 – TWO MINUTES

upavista konasana

SEATED WIDE LEGGED STRADDLE

instructions

1. Sit tall and spread the legs out to the side. You should feel a little tension, but not too much
2. Walk the hands out toward the front, gazing forward and keeping the back straight
3. If possible place the elbows flat on the ground
4. Stay here and breathe

benefits

1. Relaxes the hips and pelvis
2. Stretches the hamstrings
3. Strengthens the spine

contraindications: Neck injuries, back pain

your notes:

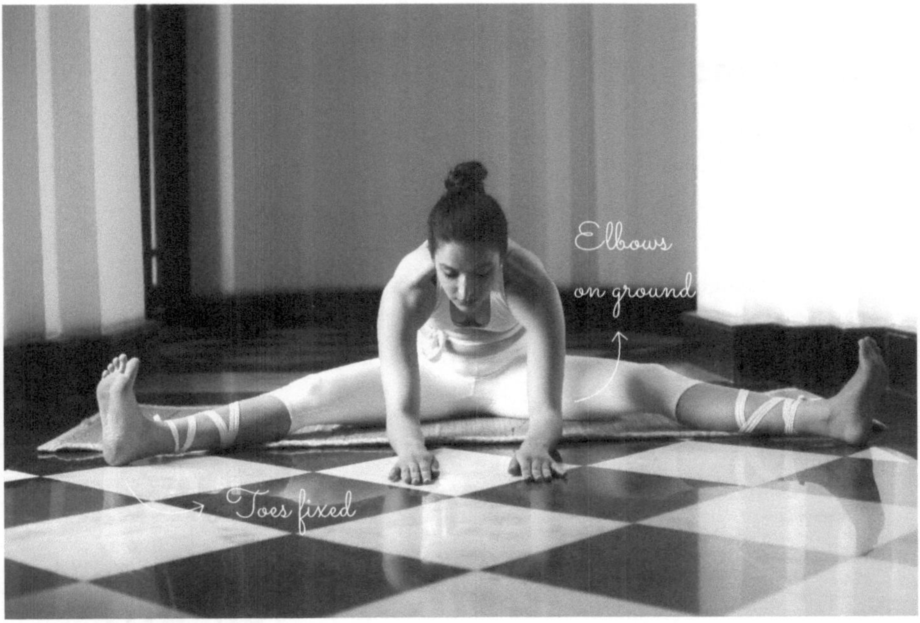
Elbows
on ground
Toes fixed

02 – TWO MINUTES

janu sirsasana

HEAD TO KNEE POSE

instructions

1. Sit in a relaxed posture with the legs stretched out in front of you
2. Bend the left leg, resting the left foot against the right inner thigh, or bringing the left foot over the right foot in half lotus
3. Inhale and raise the arms
4. Exhale and fold over gently, reaching as far as is comfortable with the hands for the right foot
5. Inhale and exhale and try to relax the body even further into the pose
6. Repeat on the left side

your notes:

benefits

1. Relaxes the spine, shoulders and hamstrings
2. Massages internal organs
3. Increases flexibility in the hip joints
4. Tones abdominal muscles

contraindications: Knee injuries, back injuries, back pain

Log out.
Shut down.
Do yoga.

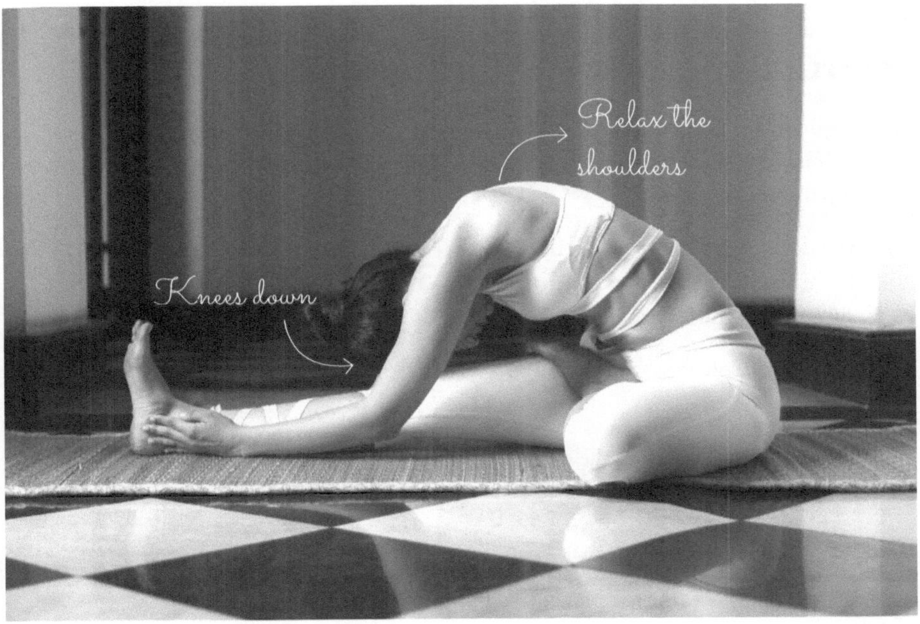
Relax the shoulders
Knees down

03 – TWO MINUTES

manjiri asana / bitalasana

CAT COW POSE

instructions

1. Begin by coming on all fours with palms below the shoulders and knees hip distance apart
2. Inhale, raise the chin and tilt the head back, relaxing the abdomen, letting it sink down, whilst raising the tail bone
3. This is the Cow Pose. Stay here and breathe
4. Exhale, drop the chin to the chest and arch the back
5. This is Cat Pose
6. Stay here and breathe for a few seconds before returning to a neutral position

benefits

1. Relaxes and stretches the neck, shoulders and spine
2. Stretches the hips and pelvis
3. Calms the mind

contraindications: None, if practised gently. Those with knee injuries can place a cushion below their knees

YOGA TIP:
When you do the movement slowly and mindfully, its effect is more powerful and meditative.

your notes:

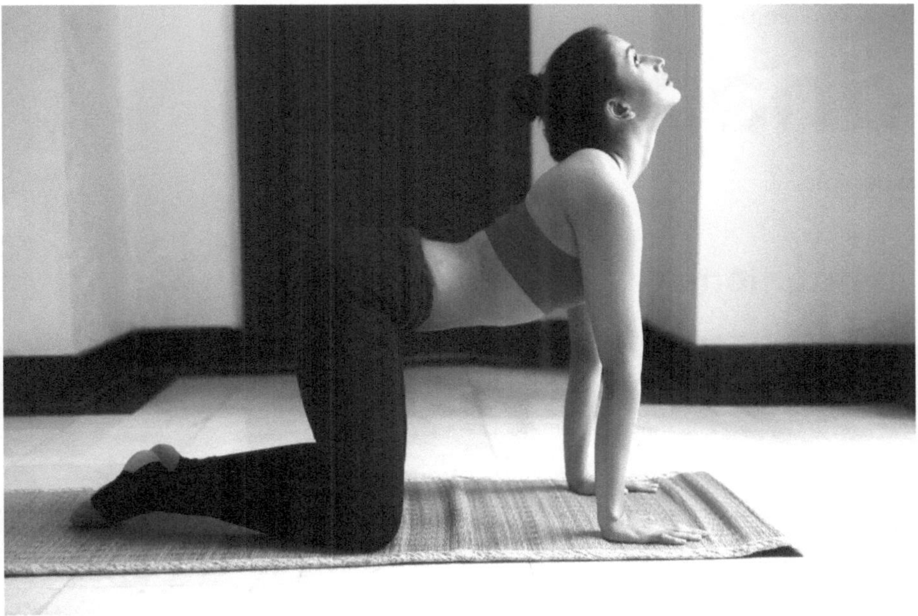

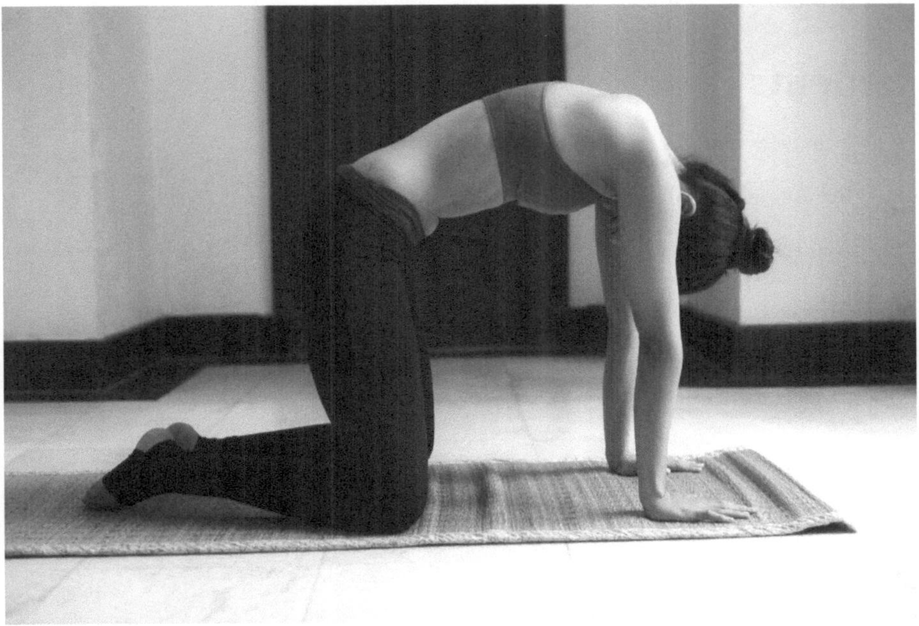

04 – TWO MINUTES

dhanurasana

BOW POSE

instructions

1 Lie flat on the stomach

2 Raise the legs and grab the ankles with the palms so the body is in the shape of a bow

3 This is Saral Dhanurasana

4 Lift the thighs off the ground. This is Dhanurasana

5 Stay here and breathe

benefits

1 Stimulates reproductive organs

2 Relieves menstrual cramps

3 Aids digestions

4 Relieves gas and constipation

contraindications: Recent abdominal surgery, pregnancy, hernias

your notes:

YOGA FACT:
If there is only *one* asana every woman should do; it is this one.

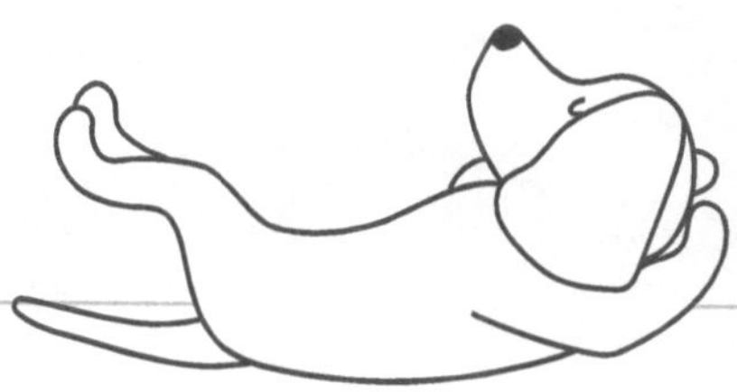

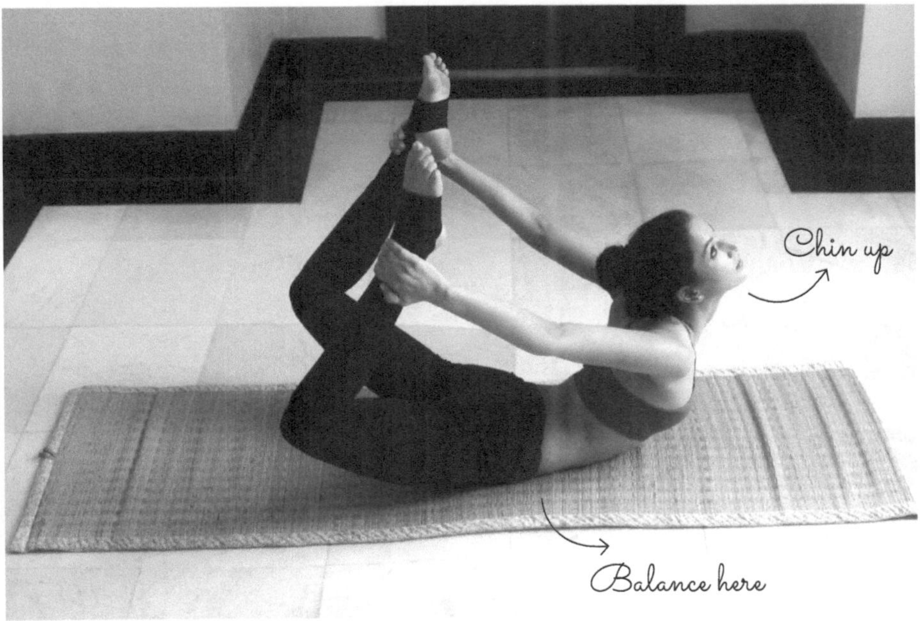

Your body will be around
a lot longer than an
expensive handbag.
Invest in yourself.

CHEST OPENERS:
The chest is an important and sensitive area for women. It is where we women store emotions, and where we hold tension. Regular yoga not only tones the chest and firms the breasts, but studies have shown that yoga also reduces the occurrence of breast cancer.

05 – TWO MINUTES

matsya asana

FISH POSE

instructions

1. Lying on the back, bring the arms underneath the body
2. Inhale, raise the chest up and place the crown of the head on the ground
3. Using the arms and elbows for balance stay here and breathe

benefits

1. Regulates functioning of the thyroid and parathyroid glands
2. Opens the chest
3. Allows for deep breathing
4. Strengthens the spine

contraindications: Neck injuries, spinal injuries

your notes:

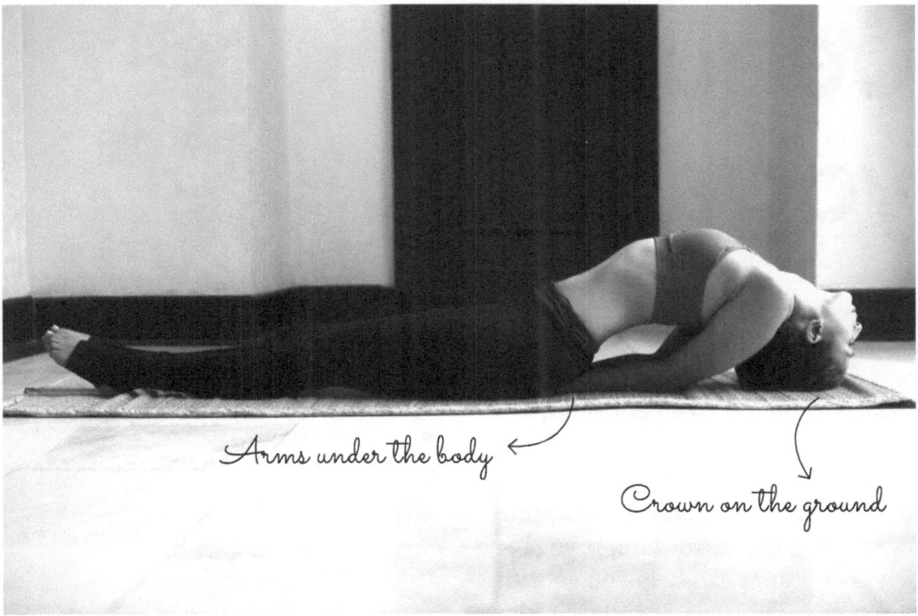

It does not matter how slowly you go as long as you do not stop.

beauty yoga

Ever wonder where the term 'yoga glow' comes from? Ever wonder why yoga practitioners typically have flawless skin? Or why celebrities, actors and models the world over take to yoga? Wonder no more. Yoga is a fabulous (and free!) way of becoming and staying beautiful. Simple yoga kriyas or asanas can help you get rid of pimples, defy ageing and wrinkles, tighten up jowls and have you shining from within. So, throw away expensive skin creams and invest in yoga instead. This 10-minute yoga sequence is the final word in your beauty routine.

your notes:

01 – TWO MINUTES
GETTING RID OF DARK CIRCLES:

cupping

instructions

1 Rub the hands together generating heat in the palms, place the base of the palms on the eyes

2 Hold for thirty seconds and continue breathing

Cupping is a simple and easy way of getting rid of pesky dark circles and under-eye bags.

The eyes are the window to the soul.

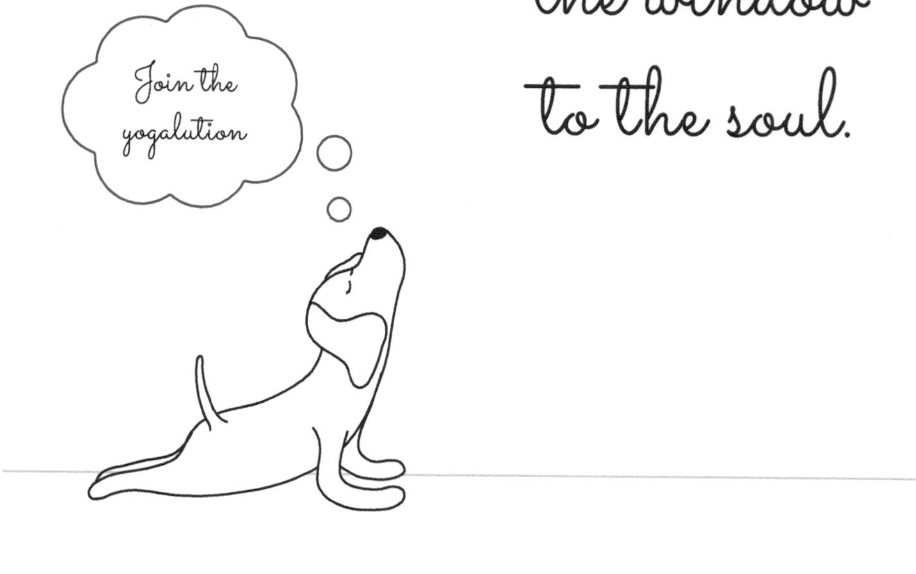

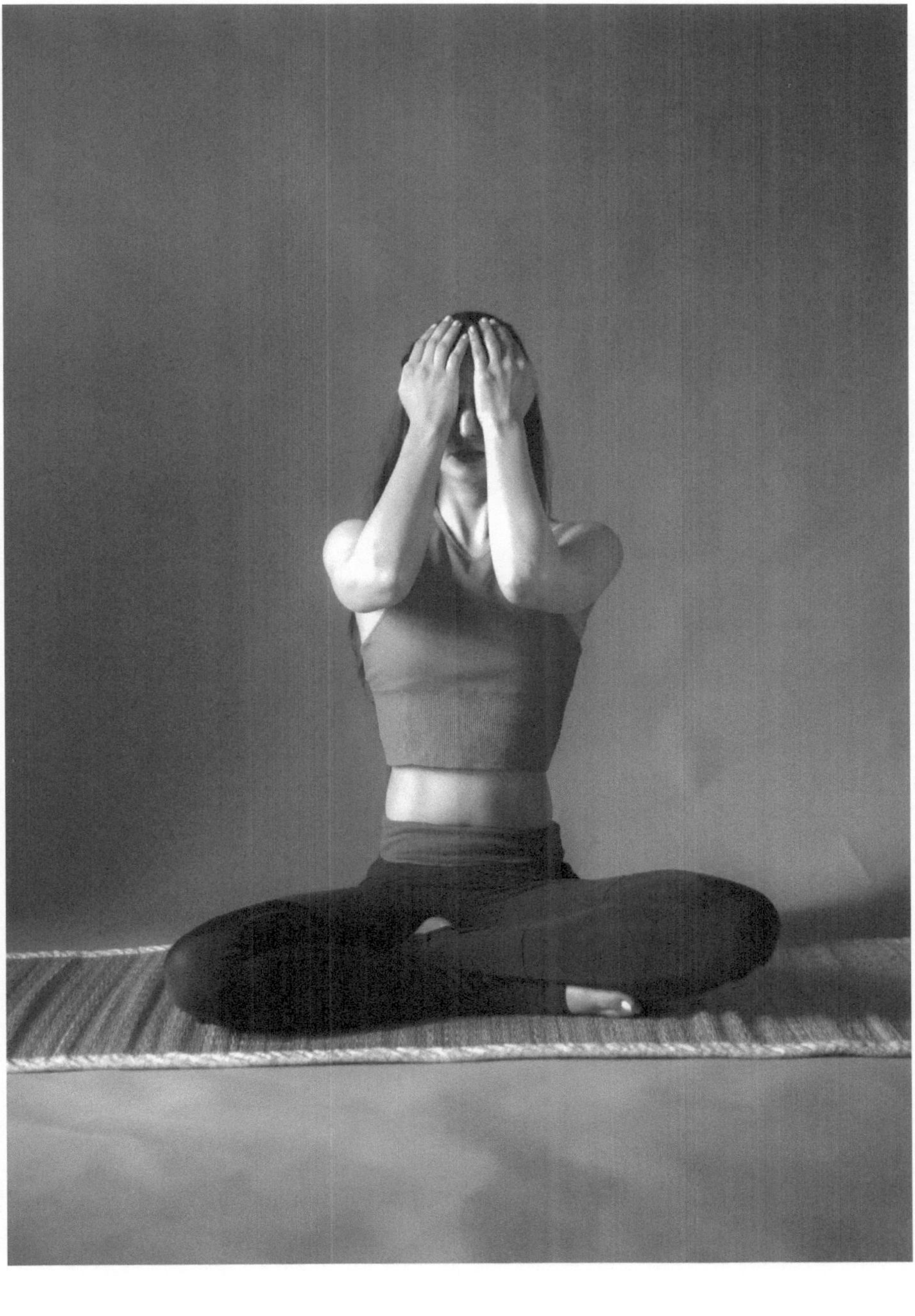

02 – TWO MINUTES
WRINKLE CONTROL:

kapala randhra dhauti

instructions

1 Rest the thumbs on the temples and with two or three fingers create a circular motion starting at the brow and sweeping around toward the nose

2 With gentle sweeping motions, bring the fingers from one side of the forehead to the other alternating between the left and right hand, i.e., sweep with the left hand fingers from right to left and with the right hand fingers from left to right. Inhale and exhale deeply when practising this

your notes:

your notes:

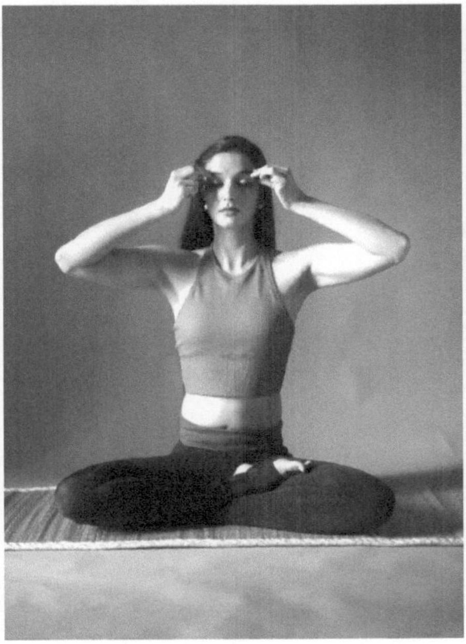 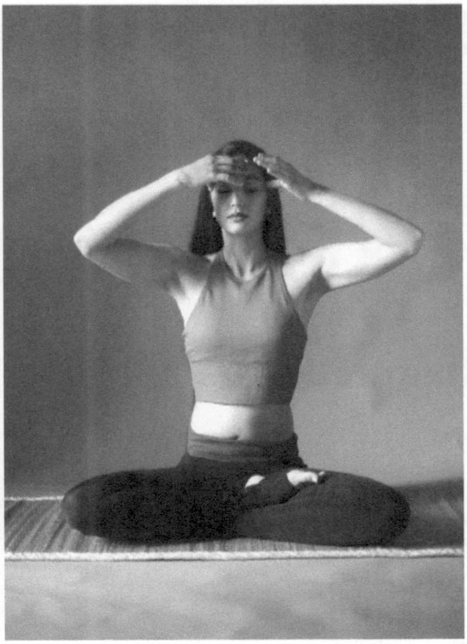

Go from a human being
doing yoga to
a human being yoga.

– Baron Baptise

03 – TWO MINUTES
SAGGING / DOUBLE CHIN:

neck exercises

instructions

1. Sit up straight in a comfortable, relaxed posture
2. Inhale and turn the head to the right. Exhale and lift the chin up and pucker the lips, pulling the skin of the neck up
3. Exhale, return to centre, facing forward
4. Repeat for the left side

your notes:

Yoga teaches us to cure what need not be endured and endure what cannot be cured.

– BKS Iyengar

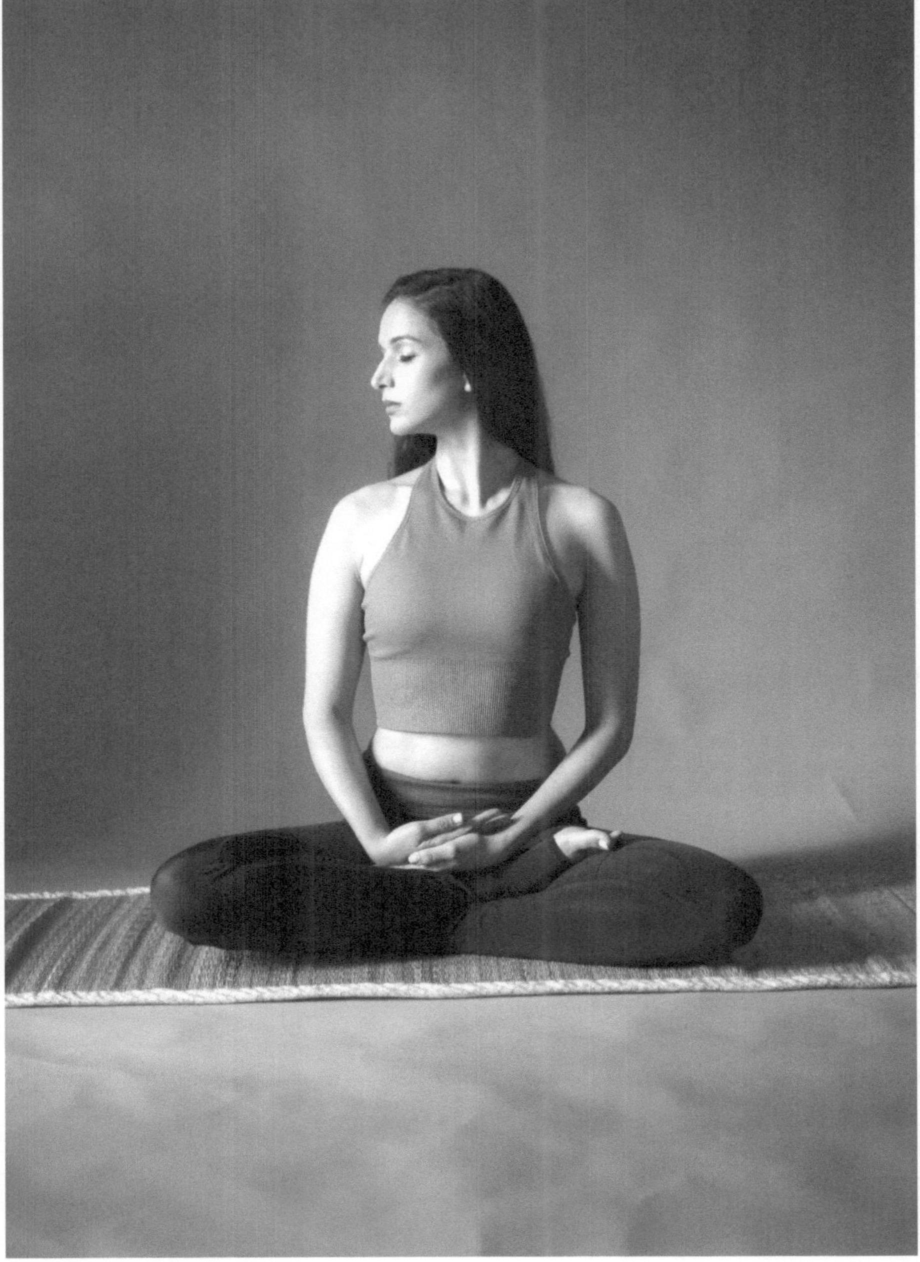

04 – TWO MINUTES

kapalabhati

REFER TO PAGE 16

your notes:

05 – TWO MINUTES

sasangasana /

REFER TO PAGE 34

sarvangasana /

REFER TO PAGE 22

viparita karani

REFER TO PAGE 200

Choose your favourite of the three.

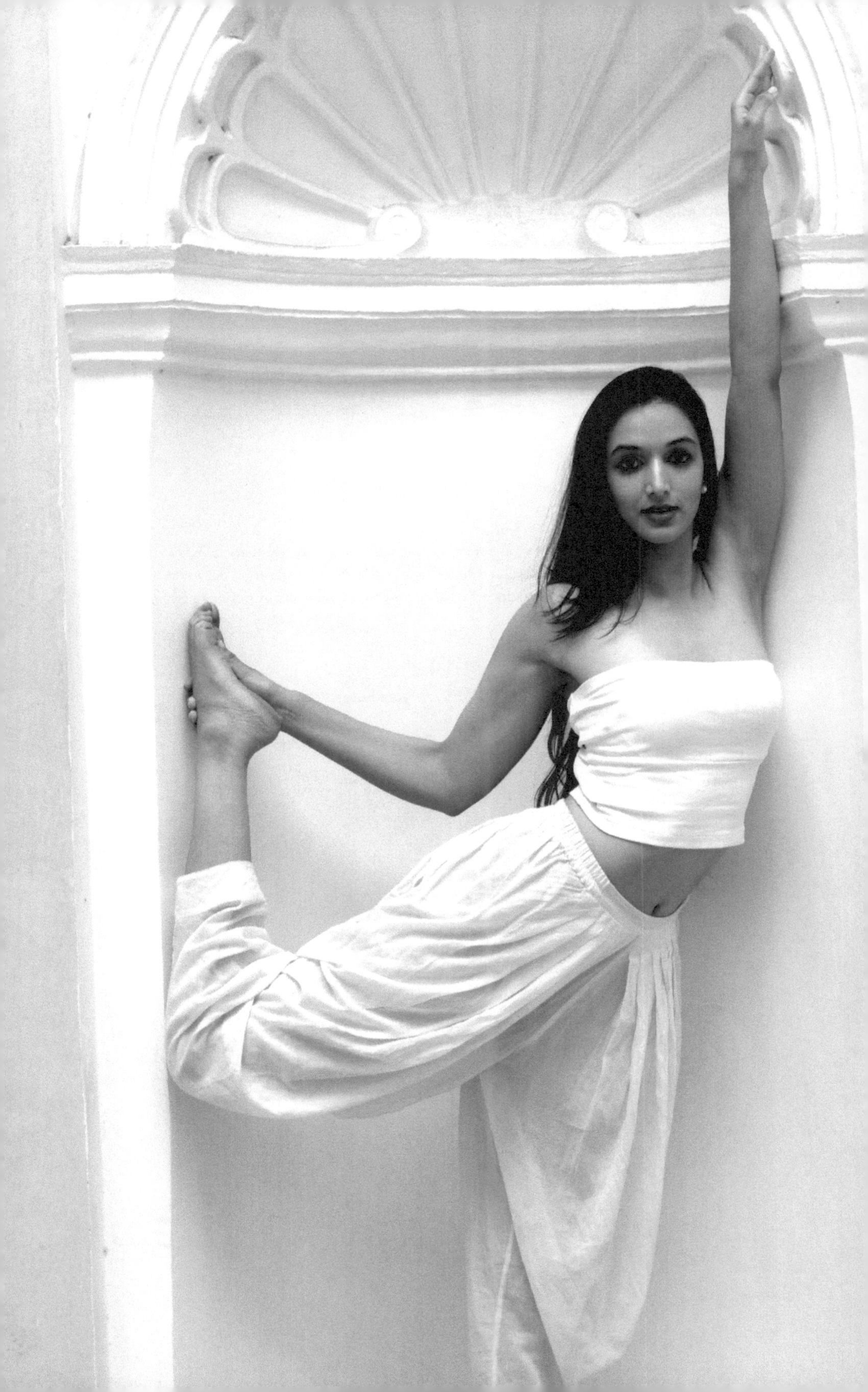

06 – TWO MINUTES

gyan mudra

HAND GESTURE

YOGA TIP:
The *Gyan* mudra is the simplest way of preventing acne and pimples. Ayurveda says pimples are caused by an imbalance of doshas – *vata*, *pitta* and *kapha* in the body. Acne usually arises due to the increase of the pitta levels in your body. Gyan mudra helps balance the pitta dominance by working on your nerves.

instructions

1. Sit up straight in a comfortable, relaxed posture
2. Join the tip of the index finger to the thumb to form the Gyan mudra. Stay here and breathe

your notes:

Be good, do good, feel good.

– Swami Sivananda

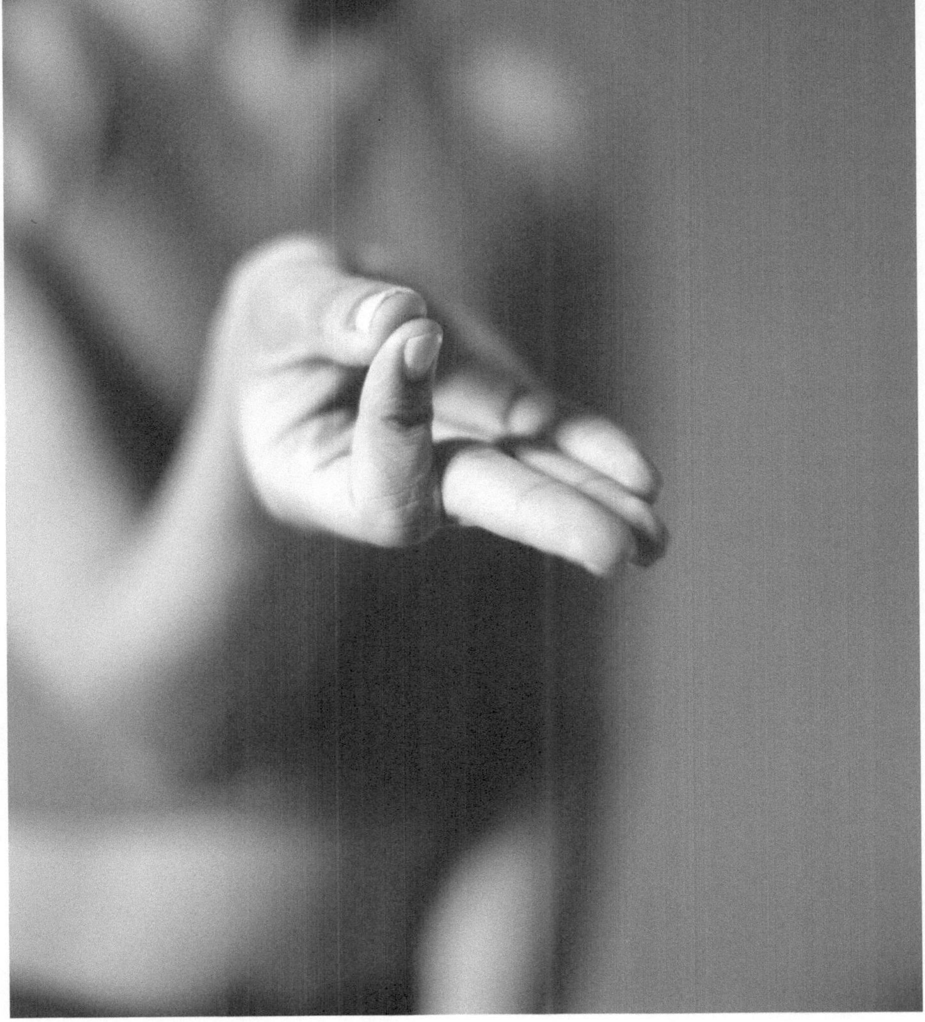

yoga for workaholics

If you spend hours sitting in a chair, staring into your computer, cradling the phone with your neck, or driving a car, you probably need yoga more any anybody else. People who spend long hours working in the office are highly susceptible to serious back and neck problems. These are also typically the very people who have no time for yoga. Start doing yoga *now* to prevent future issues. All you need is this 10-minute sequence that you can do anytime, anywhere – even *in* your office. You don't need a yoga mat, you don't need to sit cross-legged or lay down on the floor, you don't even need to take off your shoes.

your notes:

Patanjali, in the *Yoga Sutras*, says *'Heyam dukham anaagatam,'* do yoga so that you can avoid the misery that has not yet come.

01 – TWO MINUTES
BREATHWORK WITH NECK MOVEMENTS:

neck rotations

instructions

1 Sit up straight in a comfortable, relaxed posture. You can be sitting on a chair or in the car

2 Inhale deeply and twist the neck to the right. Now slowly exhale and come back to centre

3 Inhale and twist to the left, exhale come back to centre

circular neck rotations

instructions

1 Drop the chin towards the chest and rotate anti-clockwise to form a half circle. Come back to centre, facing forward

2 Repeat on the other side

your notes:

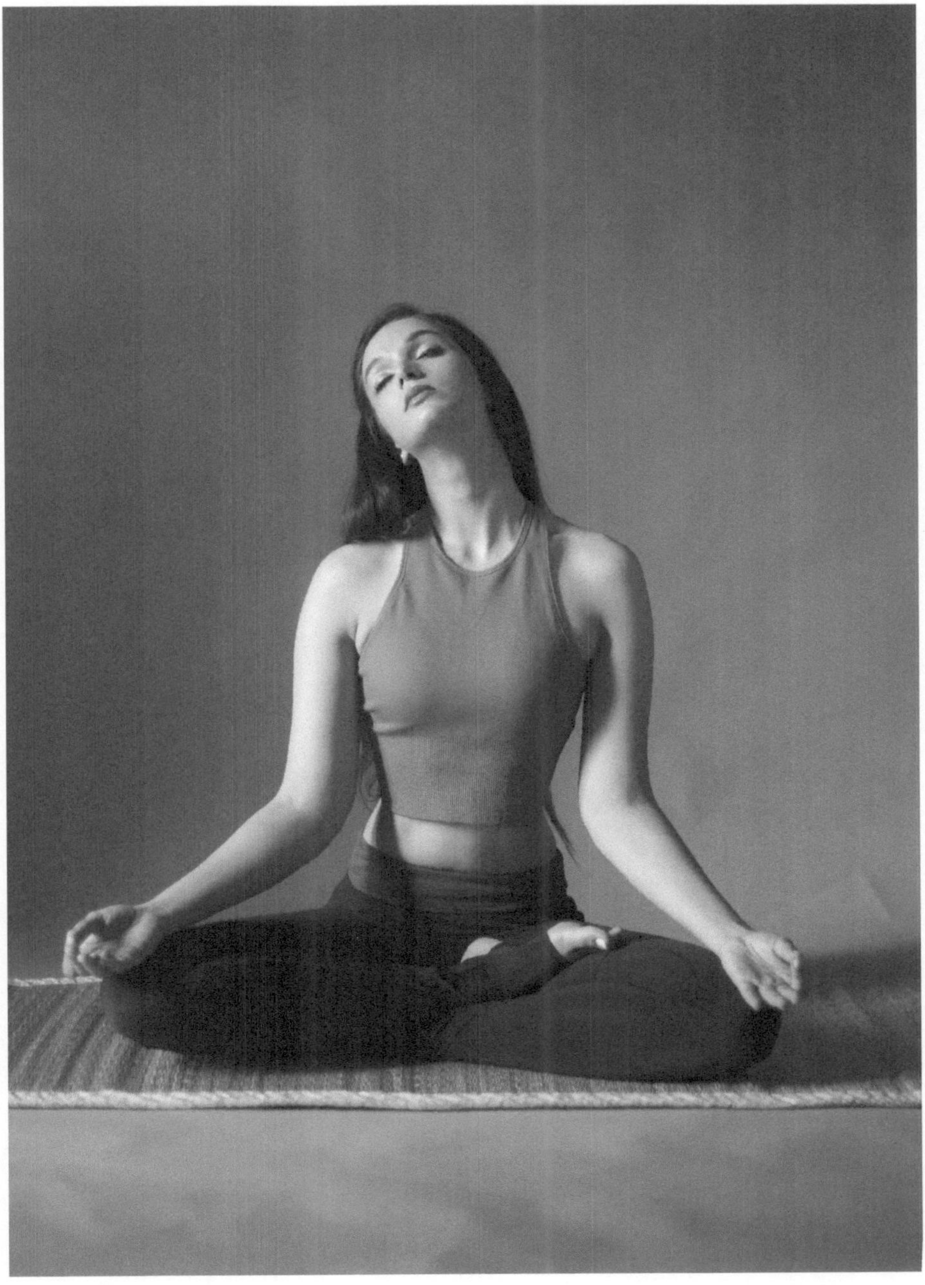

02 – TWO MINUTES

parivrtta sukhasana

SEATED SPINAL TWIST

REFER TO PAGE 18

your notes:

03 – TWO MINUTES

ardha uttana asana

TABLE TOP POSE

REFER TO PAGE 26

This is a fantastic asana for relaxing your back, more specifically your lower back, which often gets stressed from hours of sitting on a chair. You can do this with your palms rested against any table in your office.

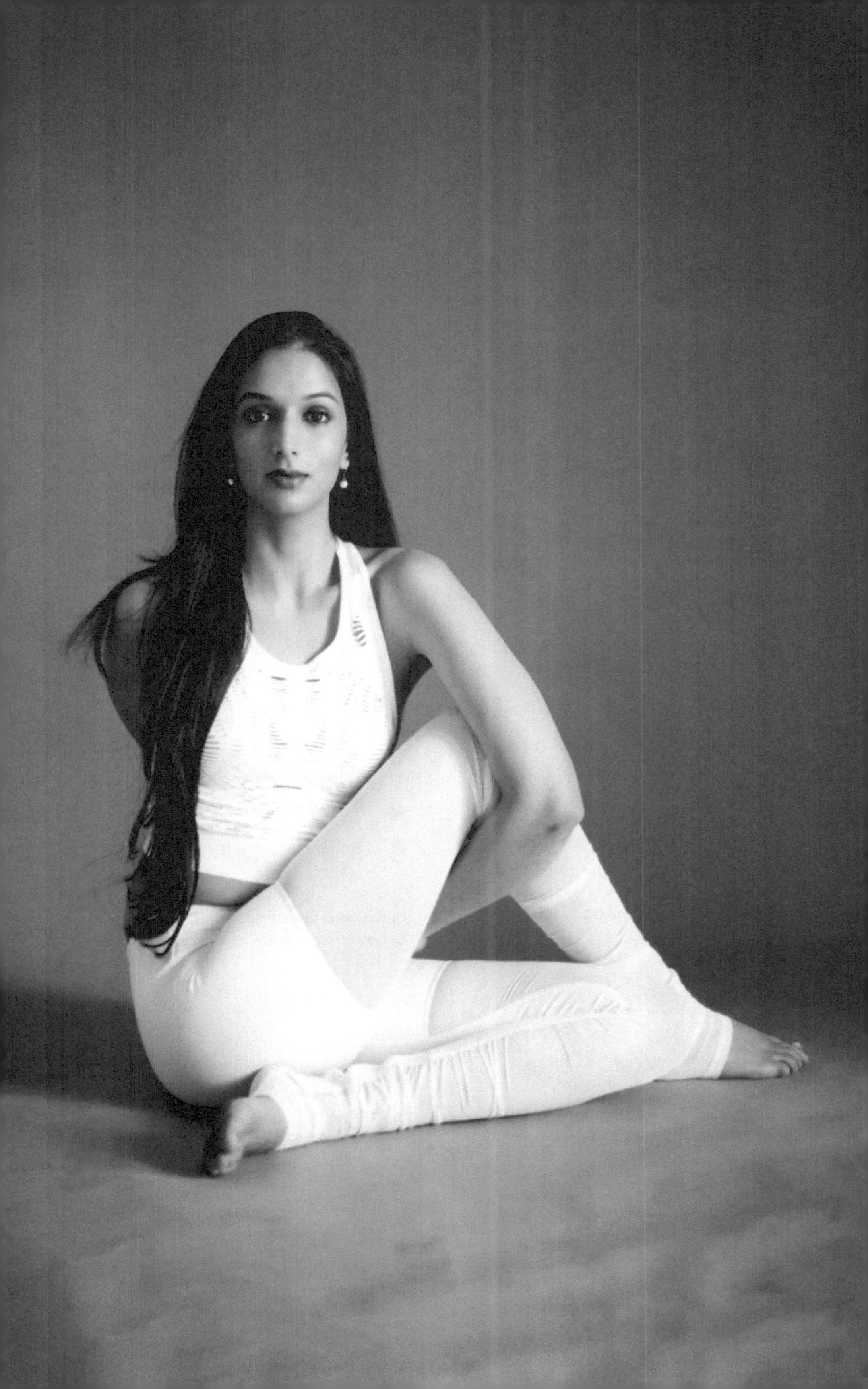

04 – TWO MINUTES

ardha chakra asana

HALF WHEEL POSE

instructions

1 Stand up straight with the feet hip distance apart and the arms on either side of the body

2 Inhale, raise the arms over the head and place the hands above the hips

3 Exhale, gently bending backwards and pushing the pelvis forward using the arms, lifting the chest higher

4 Stay here and breathe for a few seconds

5 Exhale, bring the arms down and relax

benefits

1 Stretches and tones the abdominal muscles

2 Relaxes the pelvis

3 Opens the chest

4 Strengthens the arms and leg muscles

5 Relieves tension in the back

contraindications: Spinal injuries, spinal disc herniation, carpal tunnel syndrome, high blood pressure

your notes:

YOGA TIP:
If you find it difficult to hold, you can do this as a dynamic movement.

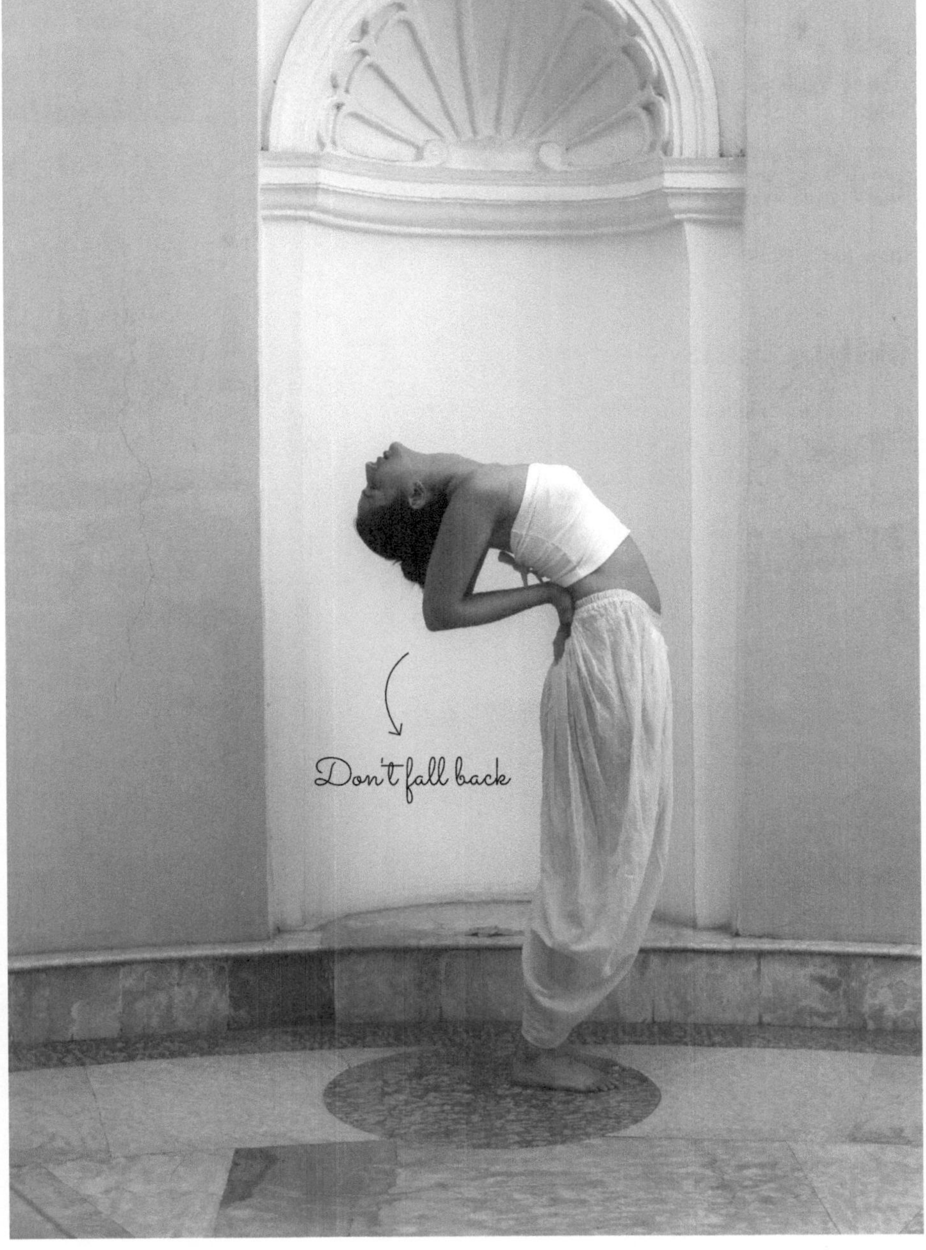
Don't fall back

05 – TWO MINUTES

gomukh asana

COW FACE POSE

instructions

1. Sit up straight in a comfortable, relaxed posture and with the feet planted firmly on the ground
2. Inhale and raise the right hand and bend at the elbow
3. Bend the left elbow and reach for the fingertips of the right hand
4. Stay here and breathe for a few seconds
5. Repeat on the other side

benefits

1. Releases tension in the shoulders and the neck
2. Strengthens the spine

contraindications: Knee injuries, neck injuries, shoulder pain

your notes:

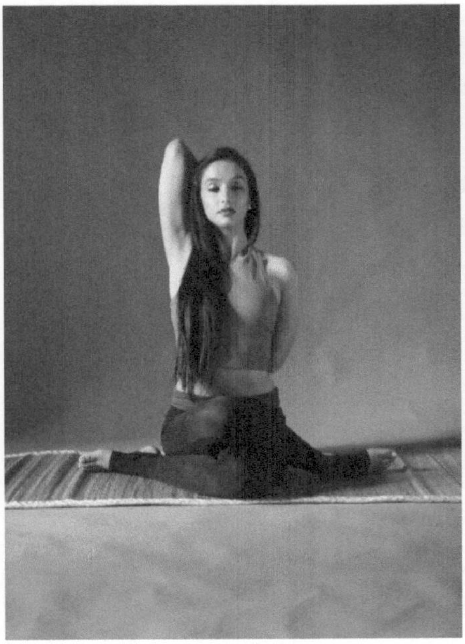

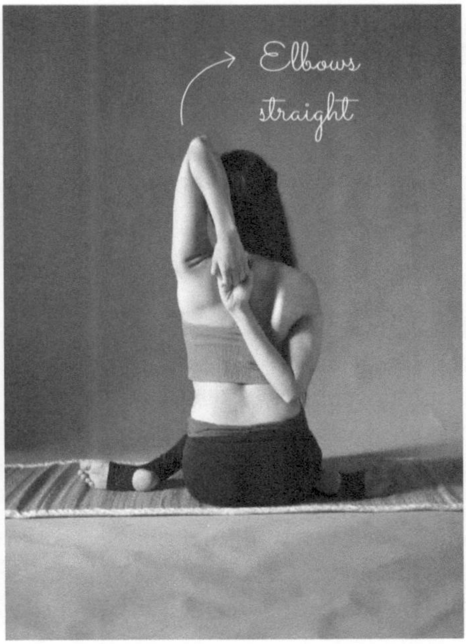

Letting go
is the
hardest asana.

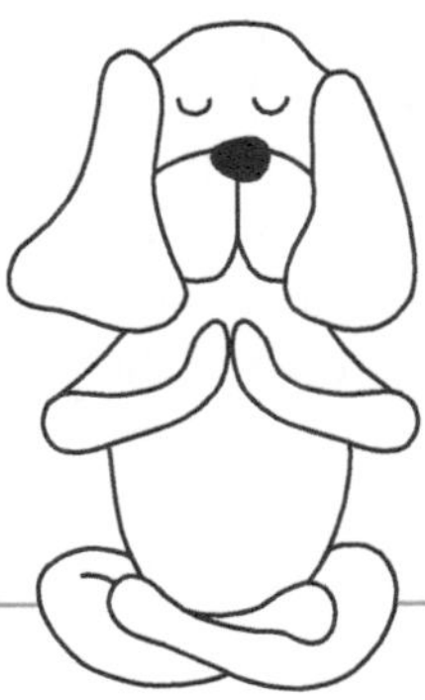

yoga to combat pollution

Exposure to harmful pollutants in the air means cardiovascular and respiratory illnesses have become synonymous with a nation on the economic rise. A decline in the quality of air has seen a rapid increase in acute respiratory infections, pneumonia, lung cancer and obstructive pulmonary diseases.

With air pollution in cities reaching an all-time high, it's more important than ever before to introduce yoga into your daily routine. Pollution related ailments like asthma are sneaky, quiet killers that are difficult to cure and can lead to chronic and fatal disease. Even a short 10-minute yoga routine will help strengthen your lungs, cleanse your nasal passages and help prevent respiratory disease. Sadly, there is much more that needs to be done to control the pollution in the environment, but in the meanwhile you can protect yourselves against it using the power of yoga.

your notes:

01 – TWO MINUTES

kapalabhati

REFER TO PAGE 16

This kriya is great for cleansing the lungs. It pushes all the stale air out allowing you to oxygenate your body in a quick and efficient way.

your notes:

---

02 – TWO MINUTES

anulom vilom

ALTERNATE NOSTRIL BREATHING

instructions

1 Sit up straight in a comfortable, relaxed posture

2 Close the eyes and take a few deep breaths

3 Begin with the right hand in Vishnu mudra with an open palm and the index and middle fingers folded down

4 Place the right thumb on the right nostril and the fourth finger and the pinky on the left

5 Closing the right nostril with the thumb inhale through the left nostril on 4 counts and close the left with the fourth finger and the pinky retaining the breath for 4 counts

6 Lift the thumb and exhale through the right nostril on 4 counts

7 Inhale from the right nostril on 4 counts keeping the left nostril closed

8 Close the right nostril and retain the breath for a 4 counts seconds, now exhale through the left on 4 counts

9 This is one complete round. Continue for 2 minutes

benefits

1 Cleans and clears the nasal passages

2 Increases oxygenation

3 Balances the prana in the body

4 Improves focus and concentration

5 Calms the mind

6 Alleviates insomnia and regulates sleep wake cycles

contraindications: None

your notes:

This is the simplest and most effective pranayama of them all. If you suffer from respiratory ailments you should increase the time that you do this practise.

Anulom vilom is typically done in the ratio of 4:16:8, i.e., you inhale on 4 counts, retain on 16 counts and exhale on 8 counts. Build up to this practise slowly and steadily. The emphasis should always be on exhaling in a controlled manner. This is the key.

your notes:

Namaste! My soul honours your soul. I honour the place in you where the entire universe resides. I honour the light, love, truth, beauty and peace within you because it is also within me. In sharing these things we are united, we are the same, we are one.

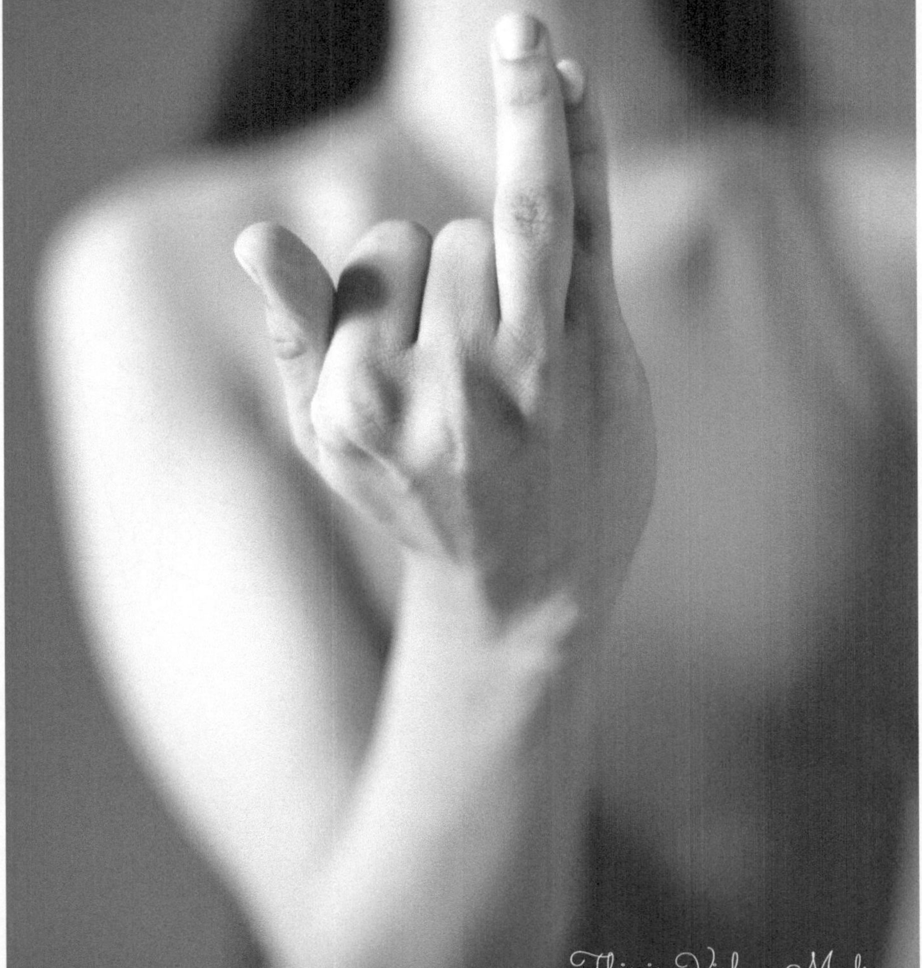
This is Vishnu Mudra

03 – TWO MINUTES

bhujangasana

COBRA POSE

instructions

1 Lie flat on the stomach with hands on either side of the chest next to the shoulders

2 Inhale and lifting the chest, bring the chin up towards the sky

3 Stay here and breathe, inhaling and exhaling deeply to open the chest

4 Exhale, and lower the chest back to the ground

benefits

1 Stretches the neck and back muscles

2 Opens the chest for deeper breathing

contraindications: Spinal disc herniation, back pain, neck injury

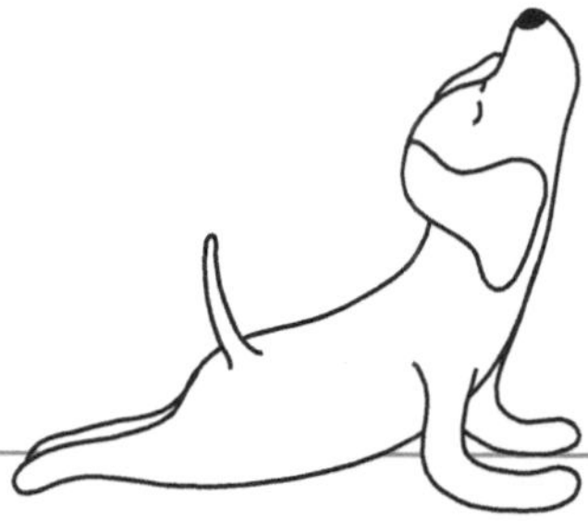

your notes:

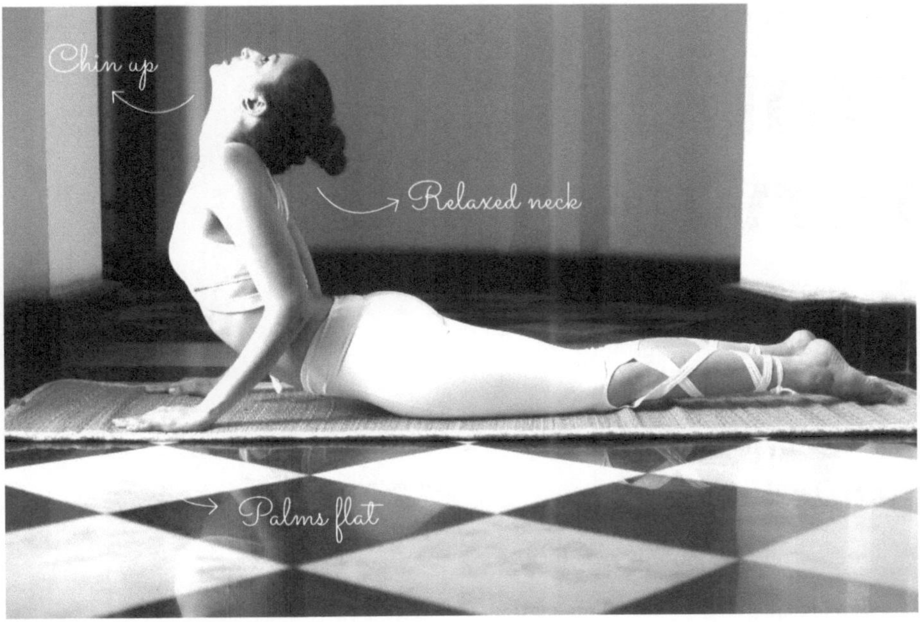

04 – TWO MINUTES

matsya asana

FISH POSE

REFER TO PAGE 50

This is a beautiful asana that opens the chest as a foundation to help prepare for other asanas. Legend has it that Matsya came down as an incarnation of Lord Vishnu as the mighty guardian of the seven seas and, in the same manner, this asana can lift you up, ground you and leave you feeling powerfully refreshed and rejuvenated.

05 – TWO MINUTES

standing forward bend

VARIATION OF PADAHASTASANA

instructions

1. Inhale and raise the arms over the head
2. Exhale and fold forward, allowing the arms to hang
3. Grab the opposite elbow forming a square with the arms
4. Allow the head and neck to hang and breathe deeply, relaxing in the pose

your notes:

benefits

1. Improves blood circulation
2. Relaxes the neck and spine
3. Stretches the hamstrings

contraindications: Lower back injuries, vertigo

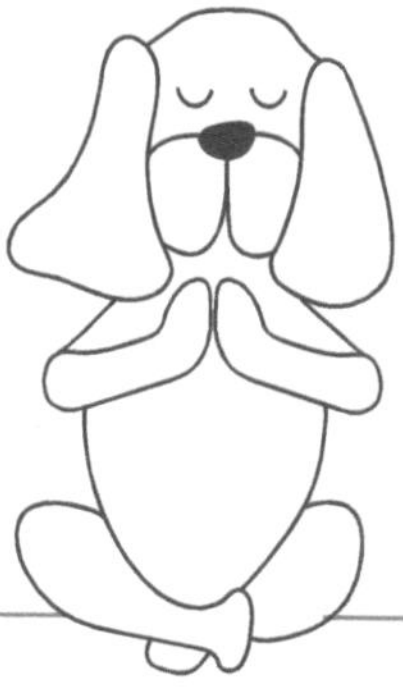

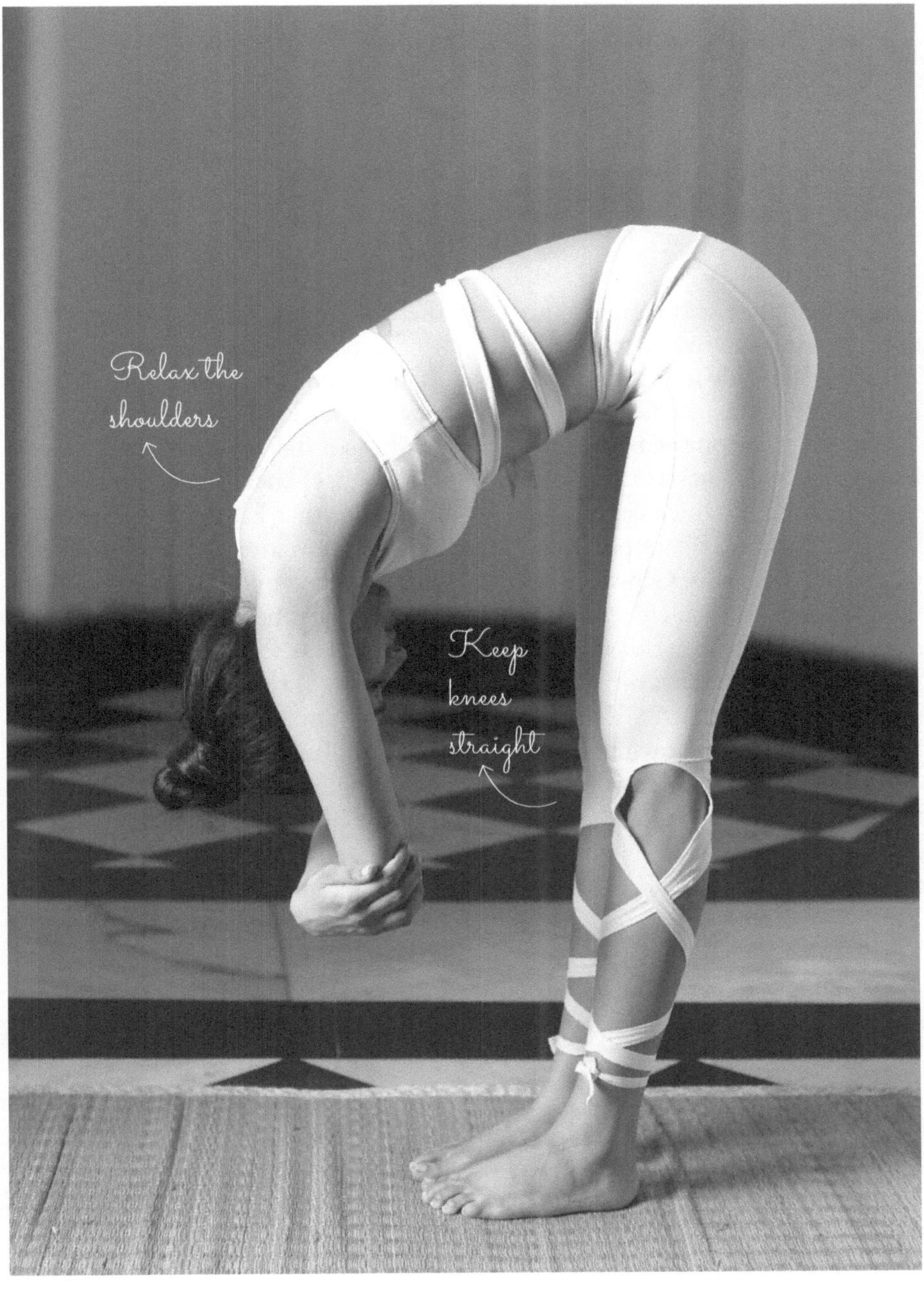
Relax the shoulders
Keep knees straight

relax, yoga and breathe

I cannot emphasize the importance of proper and systematic relaxation. Relaxing the body is as important, if not more, than exercising it. Prolonged stress on the body can lead to chronic injuries and diseases, the symptoms of which can plague you for a lifetime. I have personal experience with this. Growing up, I was both an athlete and a squash player at the national level. My priority was to always become stronger, faster and fitter. Relaxation was the last thing on my mind. I did warm ups and cooled down, but it was always done in a hurry – stretching or relaxing seemed boring and slow.

When I was twenty-five, the physical stress and strain on my body built up over years led to a terrible neck injury. There was no specific incident that triggered it. The cause was simply accumulated stress and I was advised to wear a neck brace for 3 months. At that time, I did not understand why this had happened to me – wasn't I fit and healthy? Far more than most people I knew after all? It was only when I started doing yoga seriously that I realized how important relaxation was for the body to recuperate. I learnt my lesson the hard way. But now I know that moving with mindfulness is important not just for injury prevention but also to calm the body, relieve tension and settle the mind.

This routine is best practised before you go to sleep. Relaxing your body properly ensures a deeper and more restful night of sleep.

your notes:

YOGA TIP:
The asanas below may look very easy, but remember you must consciously use your mind to relax your body. Do these asanas for 2 minutes only, but as you are doing them make sure to pay full attention with your mind and body.

01 – TWO MINUTES

advasana

REVERSE CORPSE POSE

instructions

1. Lie face down on the stomach with arms on either side of the body
2. Inhale and extend the arms out in front of the body. Now exhale and relax
3. Begin to relax the entire body starting with the toes, moving up the ankles, calves, hips, pelvis and buttocks. Continue up the back, spinal column, shoulders and arms. Relax the neck, face, forehead and head

benefits

1. Aligns and strengthens the spine
2. Stretches and relaxes the neck

contraindications: None

YOGA TIP:
A pillow can be placed under the chest to ease any discomfort in this asana.

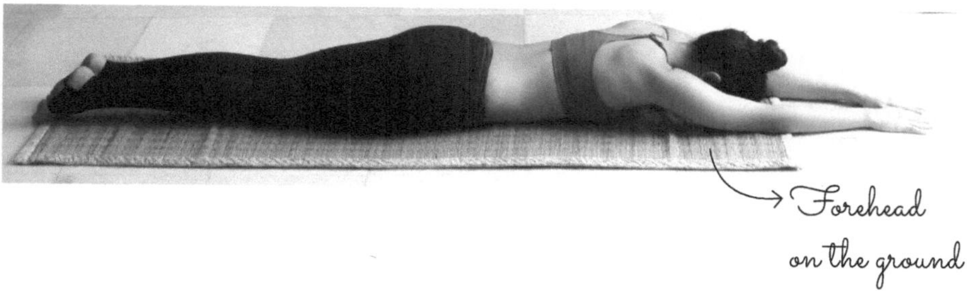

02 – TWO MINUTES

makra asana

CROCODILE POSE

instructions

1 Lie face down on the stomach with the legs slightly apart

2 Making a pillow with the hands, rest the side of the head on the hands

3 Adjust the distance of the arms for optimum comfort – if the elbows are too far out, tension will be felt in the neck. If they are too close to the body, tension will occur in the lower back

4 As you relax deeper into the asana, bring the awareness of the breath from the tailbone to the neck and feel the breath moving up and down the spine. This will activate the healing of any injuries

benefits

1 Relaxes the spinal nerves allowing for natural realignment of the spine

2 Improves breathing

contraindications: None

YOGA TIP:
Your spinal cord tends to get disfigured when the discs lodged in the vertebrae of the spine slip out of place. This asana helps in alignment of the discs.

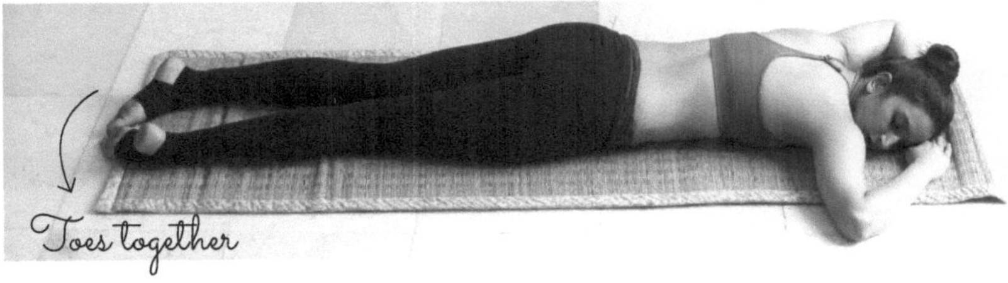

03 – TWO MINUTES

matsya kridasana

FLAPPING FISH POSE

instructions

1 Lie down on the stomach. Interlock the fingers to create a pillow, rest the right cheek gently on the hands

2 Bring the left knee up toward the elbow and shifting the position of the hands, pull the elbow closer to the knee

3 Relax and breathe

4 Repeat on the other side

benefits

1 Relaxes nerves in the leg thereby relieving sciatic pain

2 Relieves tension in the pelvis

3 Improves digestion

contraindications: None

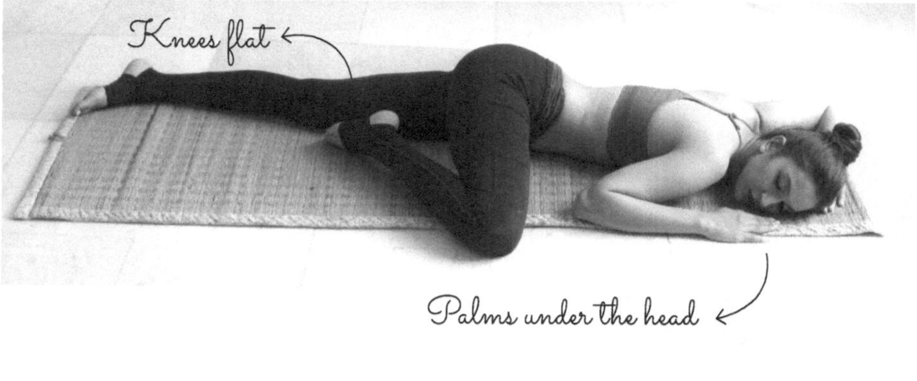

04 – TWO MINUTES

shashank asana

HARE POSE

REFER TO PAGE 32

05 – TWO MINUTES

shavasana

CORPSE POSE

REFER TO PAGE 28

your notes:

yoga for weight loss

People often associate yoga with relaxation, restoration and recovery but rarely with weight loss. The process of losing weight is synonymous with suffering and pain because who can imagine weight loss as a halfway pleasant situation? It can be, and yoga is this very way.

Cardio and weight-bearing exercises target only very specific aspects of weight loss depending on the workout routine. Yoga not only helps you burn calories and tone your muscles, it also increases circulation, promotes hormonal balance and activates digestion. These are key components for facilitating weight loss in a more holistic and long-lasting manner. The essential difference between the two methods is that yoga is focused on a shift in consciousness to a healthier way of eating and living, which leads to permanent weight control and is thus a more sustainable solution.

I used to be a gym rat. The more I worked out, the more I bulked up. I soon realized that the reason for this was that I was eating so much. Working out made my appetite go through the roof and I was overeating during every meal. Yoga controls your appetite because it harmonizes various body functions, so you will only feel as hungry as the amount of food you need to consume.

your notes:

01 – TWO MINUTES

sheetkari pranayama

instructions

1 Sit in a comfortable, relaxed posture

2 Close the eyes and press the teeth lightly together

3 Open the lips exposing your teeth. The tongue may be kept flat or folded against the palate

4 Inhale slowly and deeply through the teeth

5 After one deep inhalation, close the mouth

6 Exhale slowly through the nose in a controlled manner

7 This is one round. Repeat

benefits

1 Calms the mind

2 Improves digestion

contraindications: Sensitive teeth, dentures

YOGA TIP:
Both the sheetkari and shitali pranayama reduce hunger and thirst, so when performed, they aid in curbing food cravings or hunger pangs.

your notes:

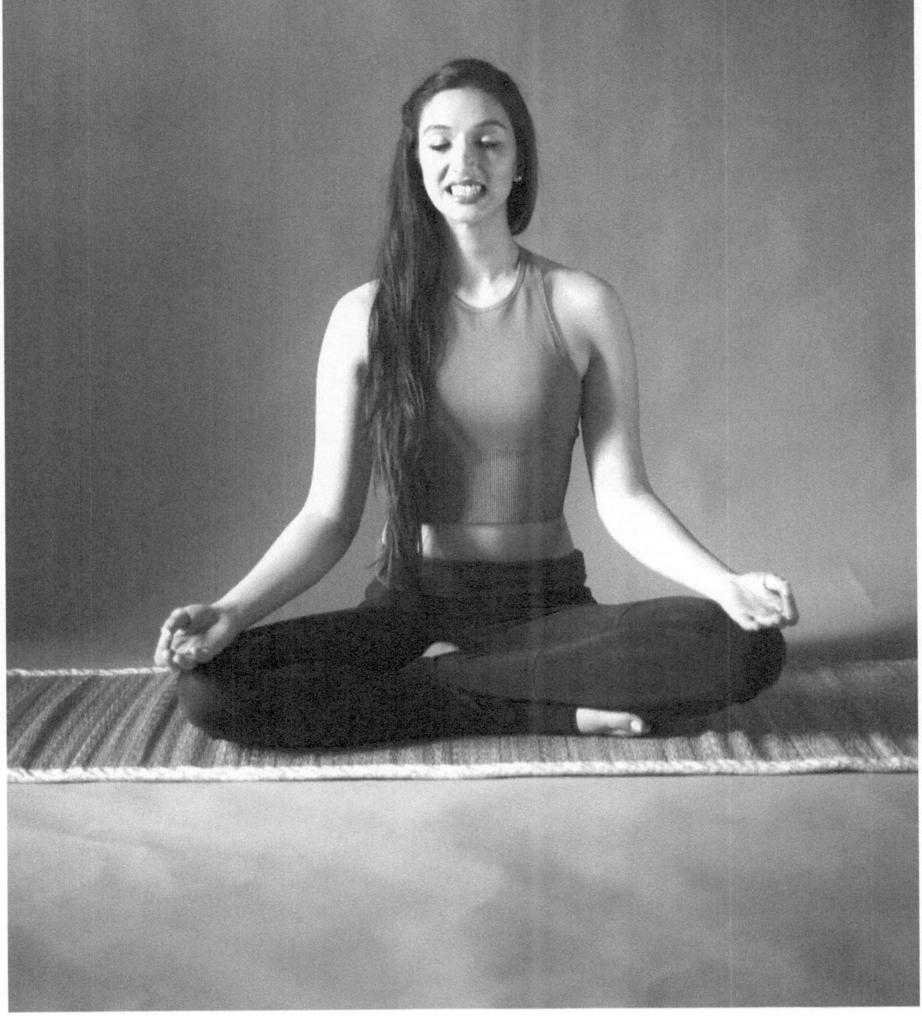

02 – TWO MINUTES

sheetali pranayama

instructions

1 Sit in a comfortable, relaxed posture

2 Close the eyes and relax the body

3 Extend the tongue outside the mouth as far as possible without strain. Roll the sides of the tongue to form a tube. Inhale slowly and deeply through the tongue

4 Close the mouth and exhale deeply through the nose. The length of the breath should produce a gushing sound

benefits

1 Alleviates hunger and thirst

contraindications: Low blood pressure

YOGA TIP:
A cold sensation occurs on the surface of the tongue and the roof of the mouth during this practise.

your notes:

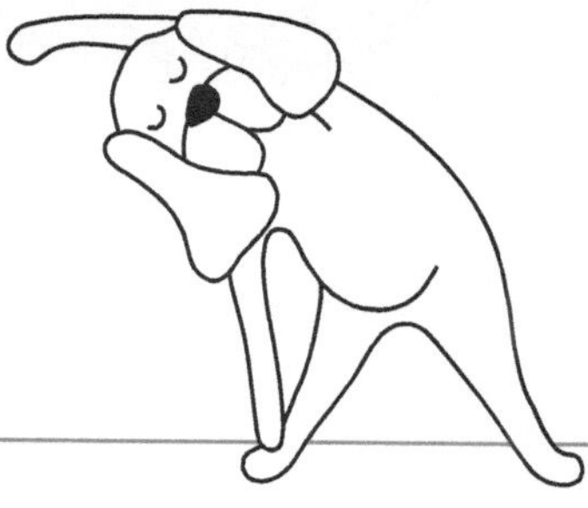

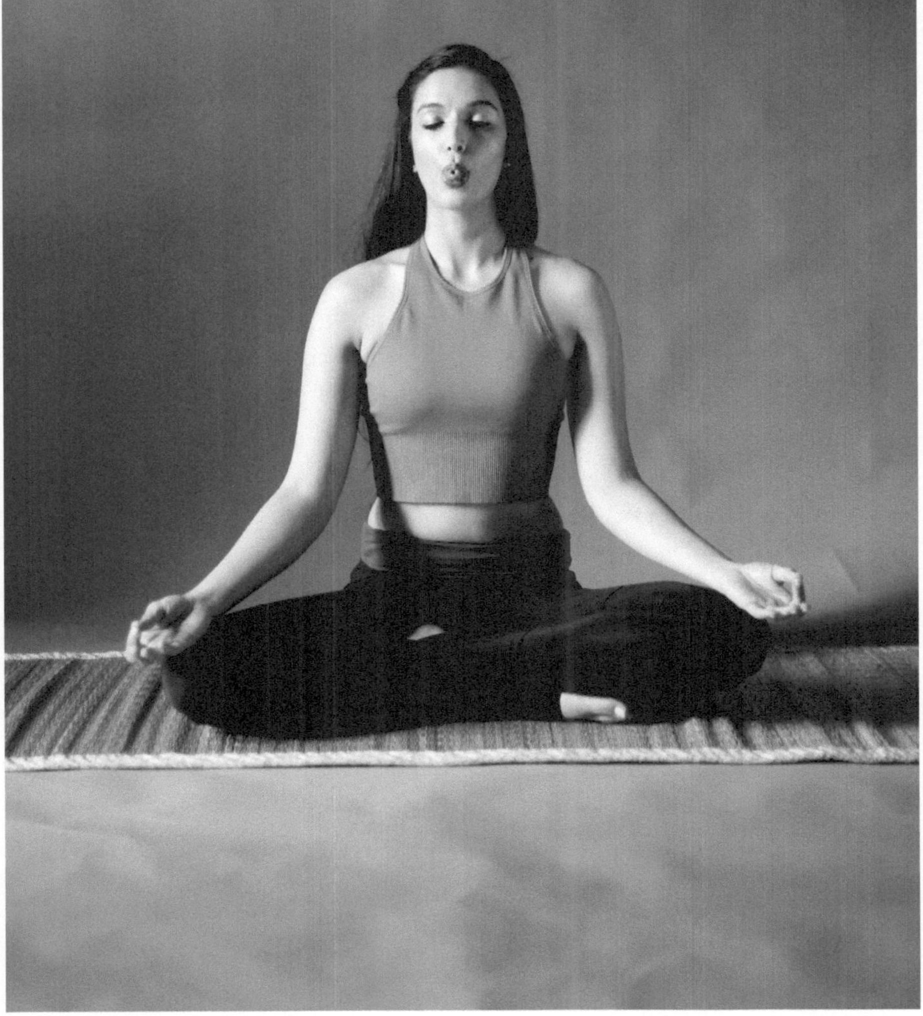

03 – SIX MINUTES

surya namaskar

The Surya Namaskar (Sun Salutation) is an all-in-one workout and a powerful aid in the process of weight loss. Sun salutations are a complete practise and this sequence of twelve postures encompasses all the essentials of asana, pranayama and even meditation. Each of the twelve postures of the salutation correspond to the twelve phases of the sun.

instructions

1 Inhale, exhale with palms together

2 Inhale, arms up, stretch back, arching the back

3 Exhale, bend down, touch the forehead to your knees, palms flat on the floor. It is best to bend the knees to protect your back in this posture

4 Inhale, right leg back, palms in line with the feet, chin up pointing to the sky

5 Retain the breath and bring the right leg back in plank position

6 Exhale, go down, chin down, chest down, knees down, hips up

7 Inhale, come up in Cobra or Bhujangasana, elbows pointed out, toes pointed out

8 Exhale, inverted V

9 Inhale, right leg forward in line with your palm, chin pointing up to the sky

10 Exhale, bring the left leg forward and bring your forehead to the knees, palms flat on the floor

11 Inhale, arms up, stretch up, arching back

12 Exhale, bring the arms down

13 Repeat the same now on the left side, replacing all instructions for the right leg with the left leg

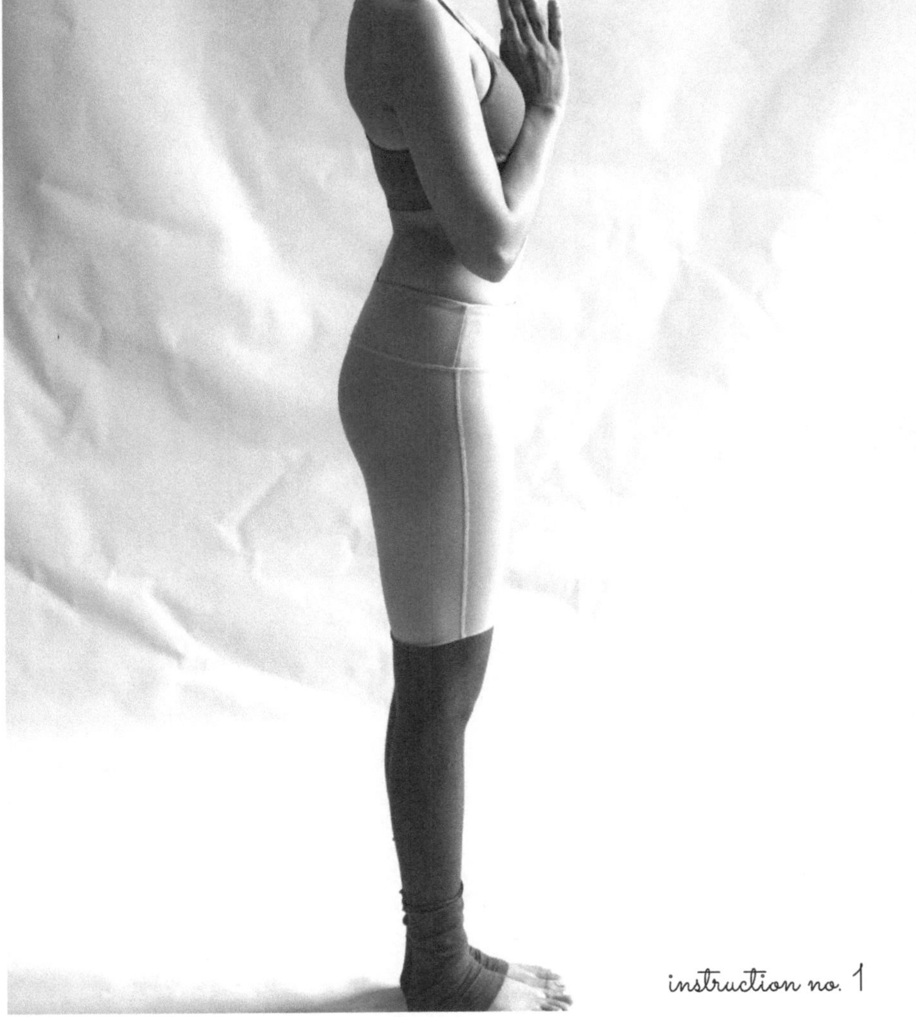

instruction no. 1

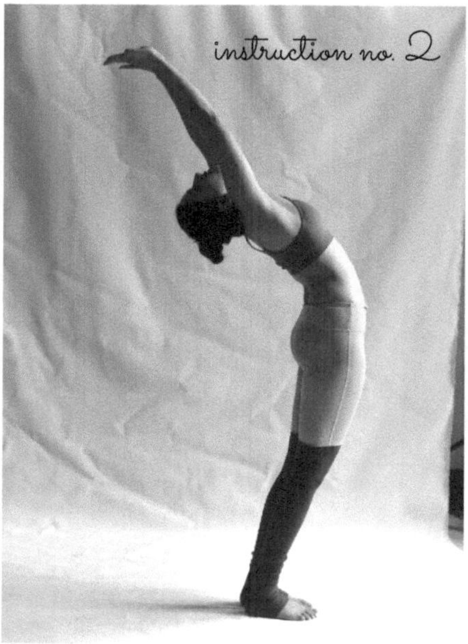

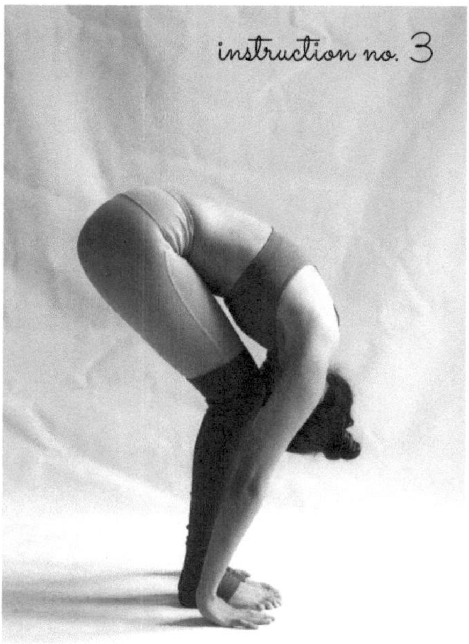

benefits

1 Stretches and strengthens the spine, legs, arms, back and shoulders

2 Balances irregular breathing and heart rate, reduces stress

3 Improves blood circulation in the body

4 Full body workout

contraindications: Fever, acute inflammation, blood toxicity, high blood pressure, spinal disc herniation, back pain, recent surgery

your notes:

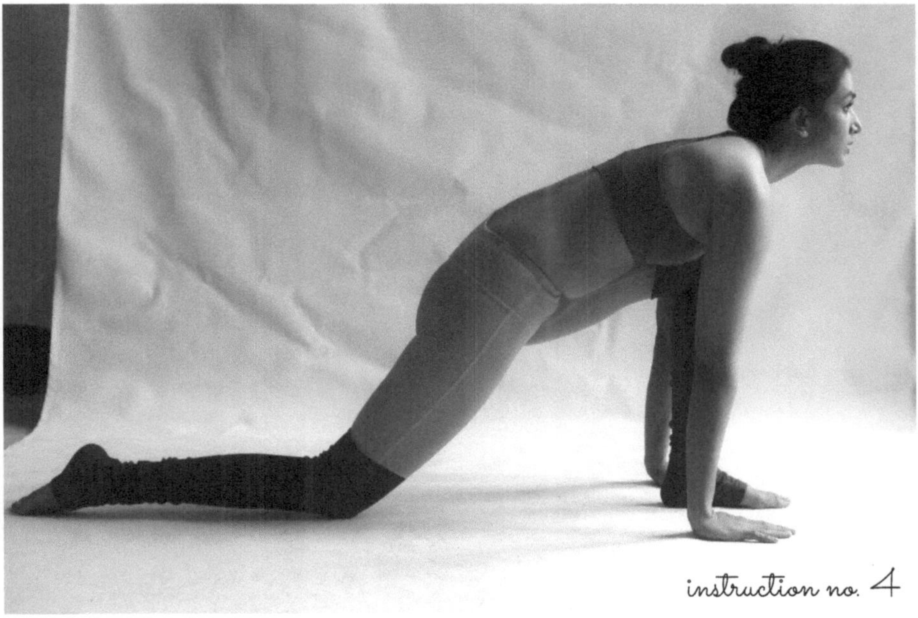

instruction no. 4

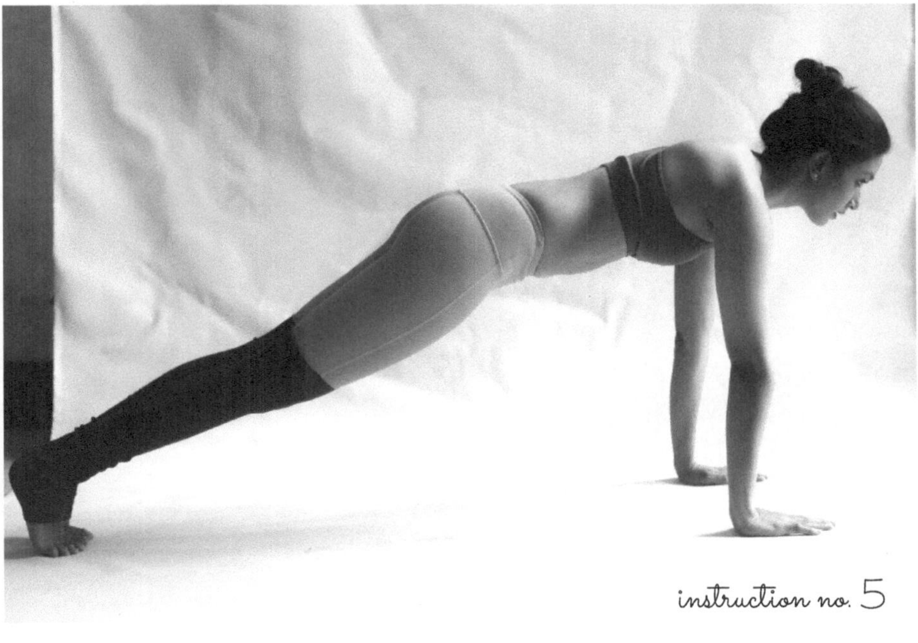

instruction no. 5

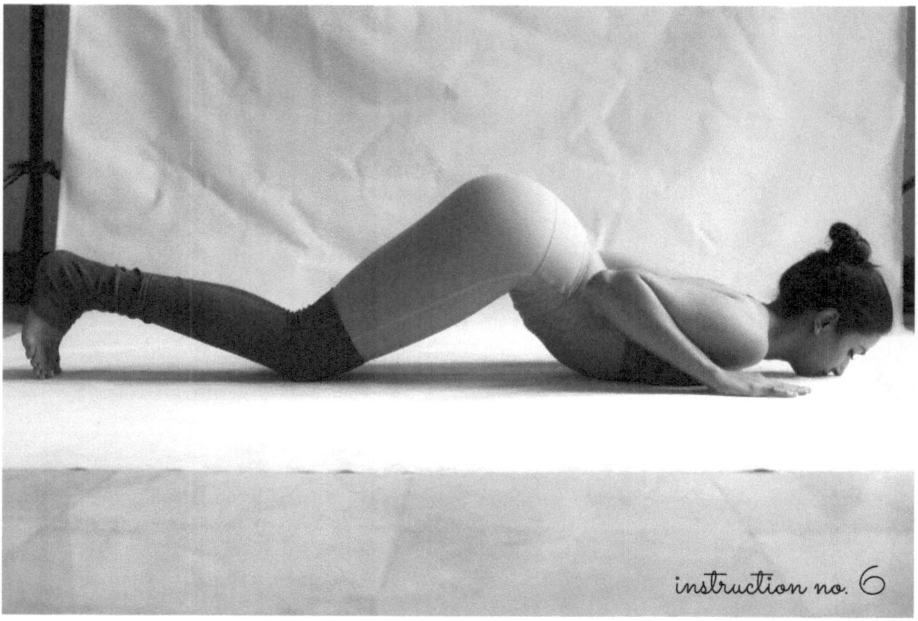

instruction no. 6

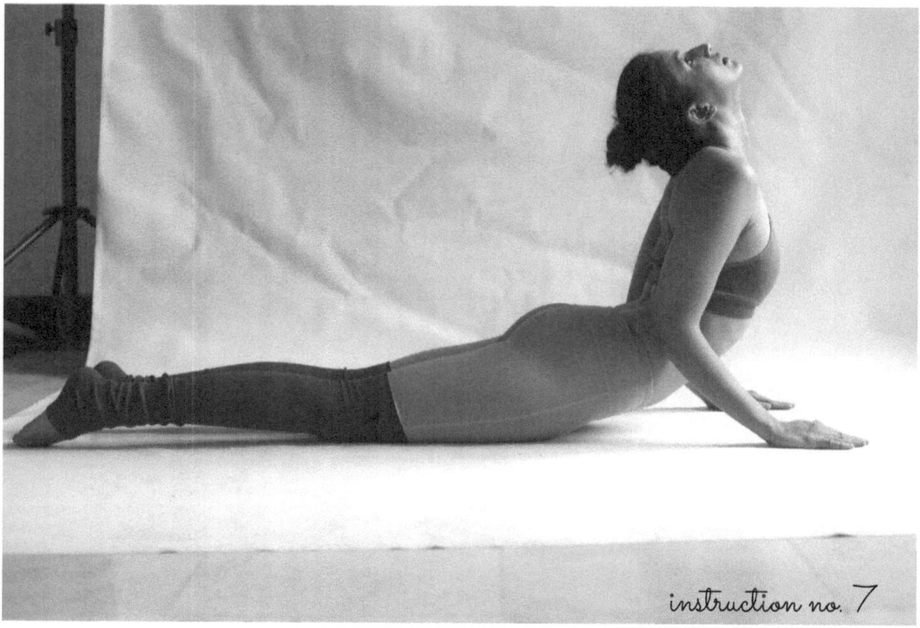

instruction no. 7

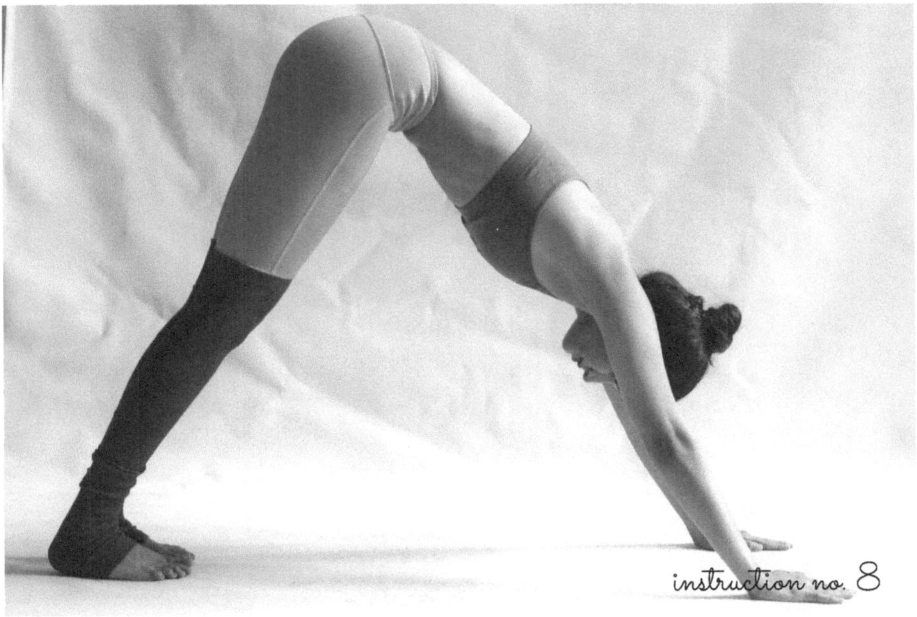
instruction no. 8

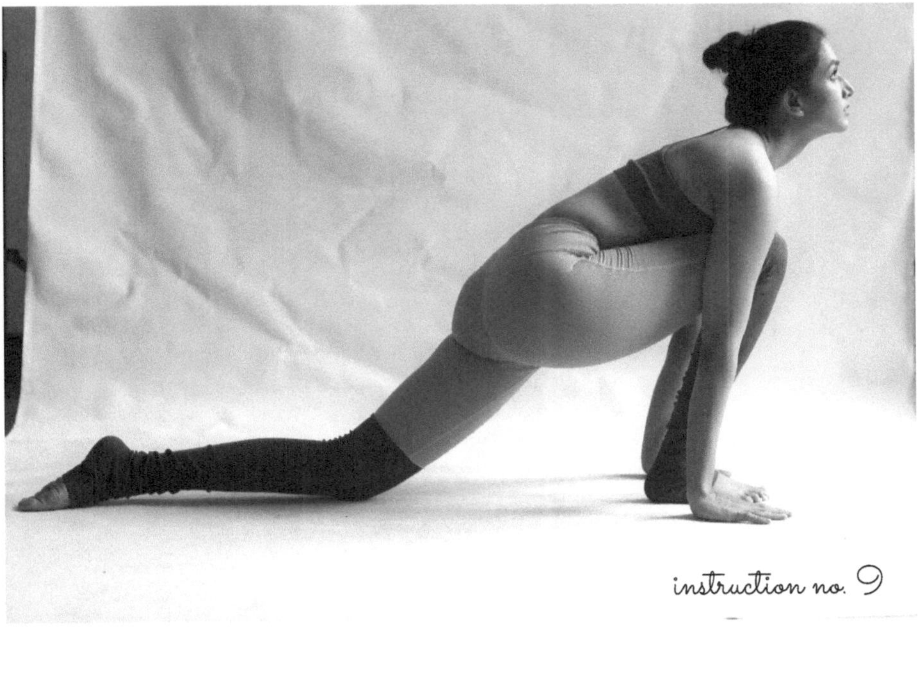
instruction no. 9

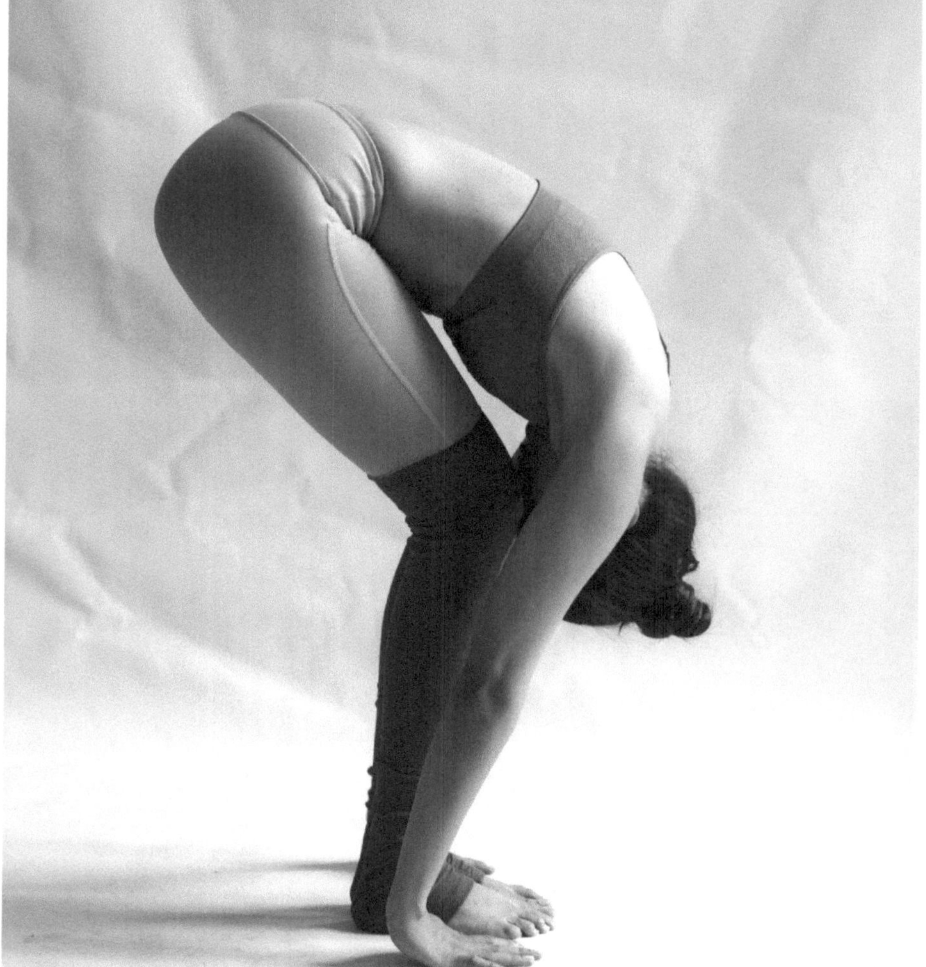

instruction no. 10

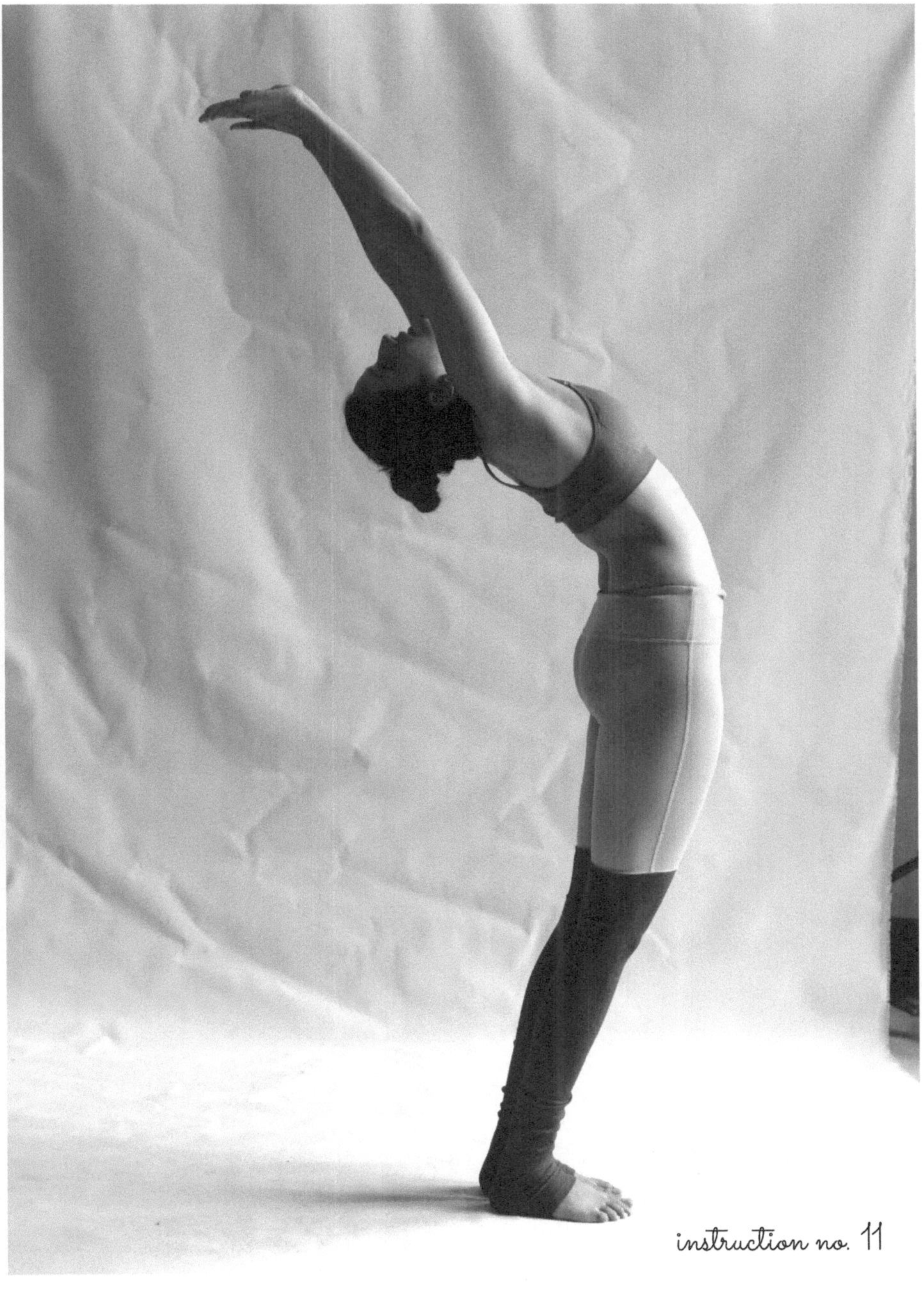

instruction no. 11

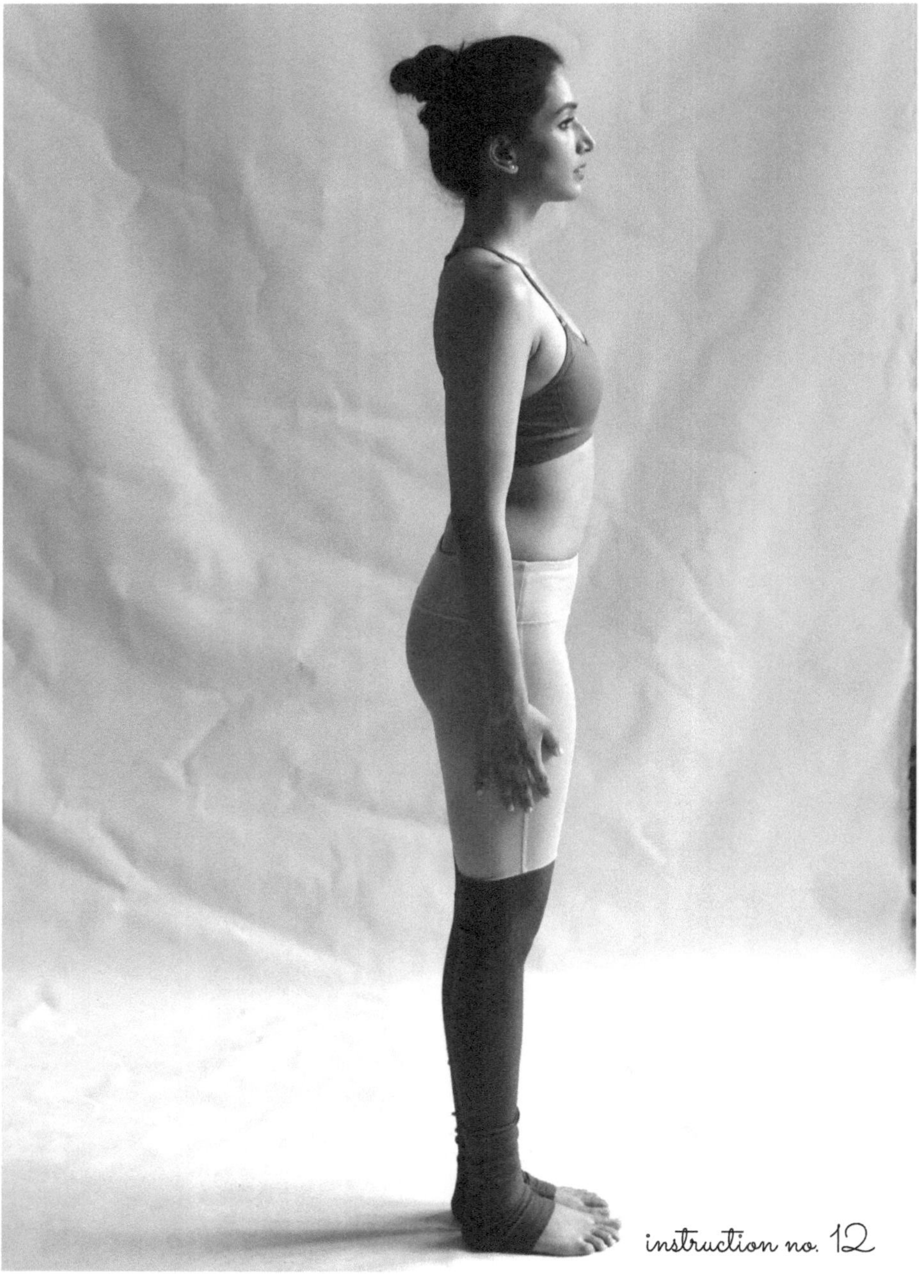

instruction no. 12

YOGA TIP:
During surya namaskar, it is critical to breathe along with the movements. When you bring the chest up you inhale, when you bring the chest down, you exhale and when you are in neutral position you retain the breath.

Inhale.
Exhale.
Breathe.

your notes:

04 – THIRTY SECONDS

adho mukha svanasana

DOWNWARD DOG

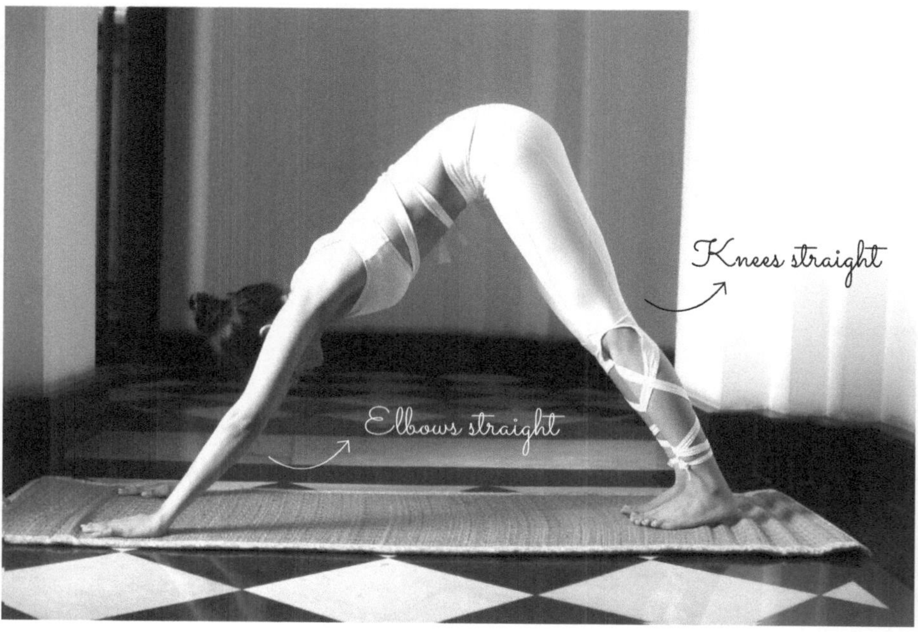

instructions

1 Begin on all fours with the palms and knees on the ground

2 Inhale and raise the hips, pressing into the ground firmly with the palms and feet

3 As you inhale and exhale relax and go deeper into the pose

benefits

1 Improves posture

2 Strengthens the spine, arms, wrists

3 Stretches chest and lungs, shoulders, and abdomen

4 Massages abdominal organs

5 Stimulates internal detox

contraindications: Back injury, carpal tunnel syndrome, migraines

your notes:

Losing your balance is normal, trying again is what makes you a yogi.

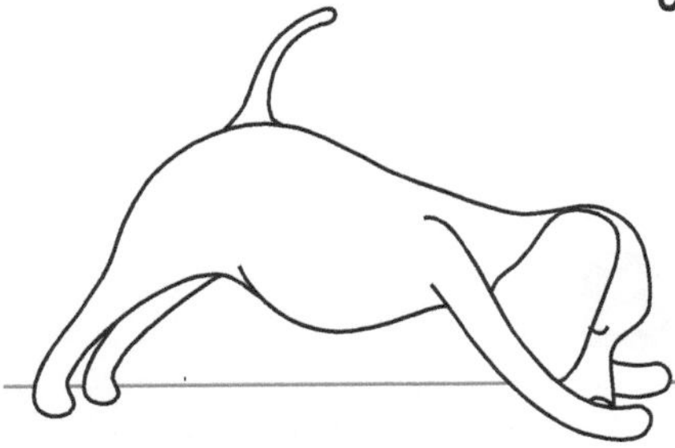

05 – TWO MINUTES

anjaneyasana

CRESCENT MOON POSE

instructions

1. Stand on the mat with the feet 3-4 feet comfortably apart and raise the arms up so they are perpendicular to the floor and parallel to each other
2. Bend the right knee so that it is parallel to the ground, keeping the left leg straight
3. Inhale and reach up to the sky with the arms, expanding the chest and arching the back
4. With every inhalation reach higher toward the sky, and with every exhalation sink deeper into the pose with the hips
5. Repeat on the left side

benefits

1. Stabilizes muscles in the legs and feet
2. Improves balance and concentration
3. Strengthens the core
4. Improves digestion

contraindications: Circulatory diseases, high blood pressure, respiratory disorders

your notes:

06 – TWO MINUTES

shavasana

CORPSE POSE

REFER TO PAGE 28

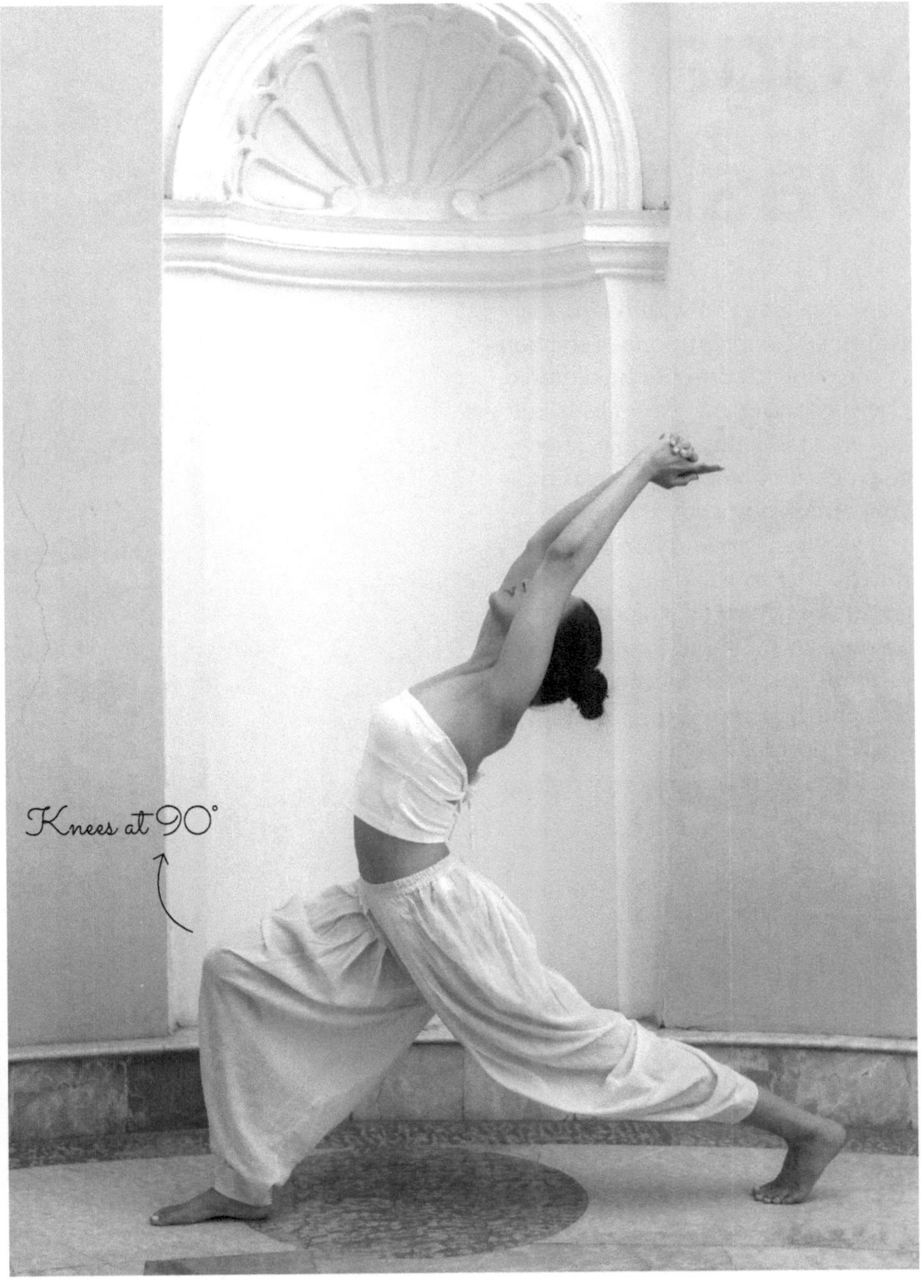
Knees at 90°

yoga for washboard abs

Can yoga give you washboard abs? Absolutely, and with only a fraction of the effort that would be required elsewhere. Getting great abs is not just about burning fat, it is about getting rid of bloating, increasing your circulation and metabolism and about improving hormonal functioning so you don't gain unnecessary weight. Yoga works on these at the same time, making your abs strong both inside and out. Remember what's going on inside is as important as what's going on outside. This is the only way to long-term health!

your notes:

01 – TWO MINUTES

kapalabhati

REFER TO PAGE 16

The muscular action generated by Kapalabhati is the equivalent of doing crunches or sit-ups at the gym. The pumping action from rapid inhalation and exhalation leads to a more toned abdomen. More importantly, this kriya helps massage the internal organs and has a detoxifying effect on the body.

benefits

1 Improves blood circulation

2 Increases oxygenation

3 Strengthens the lungs

4 Stimulates the digestive organs

5 Tones the abdominal muscles

contraindications: Respiratory diseases, circulatory diseases, epilepsy, hernias, gastric ulcers

note: This kriya is not recommended during the first 3 months of pregnancy

your notes:

Relax, Yoga, Breathe.

02 – TWO MINUTES

chakki chalanasana

MILL CHURNING POSE

instructions

1. Sit in a comfortable, relaxed position
2. Clasp the hands and stretch the arms out in front of you
3. Inhale and start moving the upper part of your body to the front and right, forming an imaginary circle with the body
4. Exhale as you go backward and to the left
5. Keep breathing slowly and deeply while rotating. Complete 5-10 rounds in one direction and then repeat on the other side

benefits

1. Tones abdominal muscles
2. Relaxes the pelvic area

contraindications: Pregnancy, low blood pressure, lower back pain, recent abdominal surgeries, neck injuries

your notes:

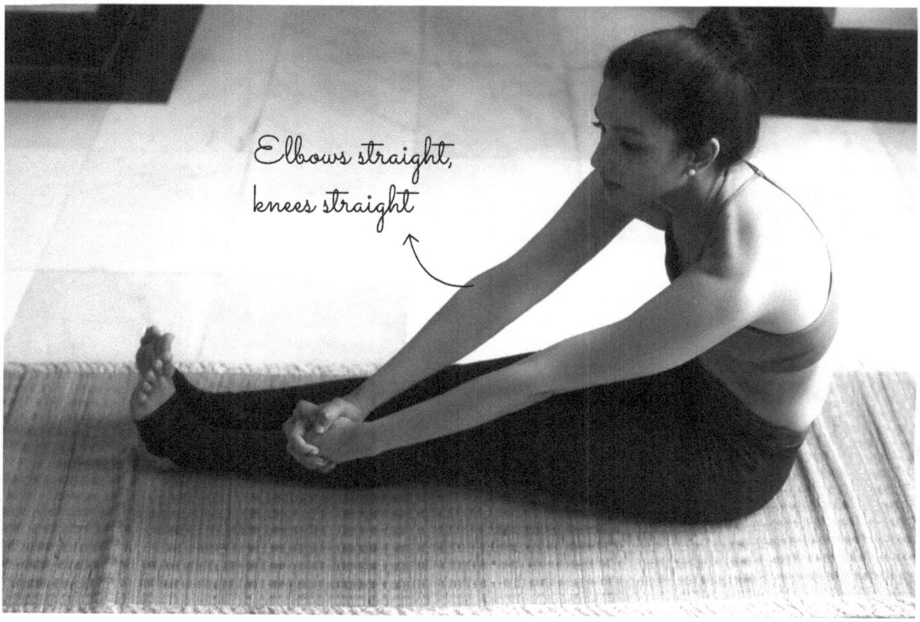

03 – TWO MINUTES

janu sirsasana

HEAD TO KNEE POSE

REFER TO PAGE 44

your notes:

04 – TWO MINUTES

halasana

PLOW POSE

instructions

1. Lie flat on the back with arms on either side of the body
2. With controlled momentum swing the legs over the head
3. Placing the palms firmly on the ground inhale and exhale, deeply reaching for the ground with the feet as far as possible. If your feet reach the ground, clasp your palms

benefits

1. Activates digestion
2. Strengthens the abdominal muscle
3. Regulates the thyroid gland
4. Reduces stress and fatigue

contraindications: Spinal injuries, back injuries, neck injuries, high blood pressure

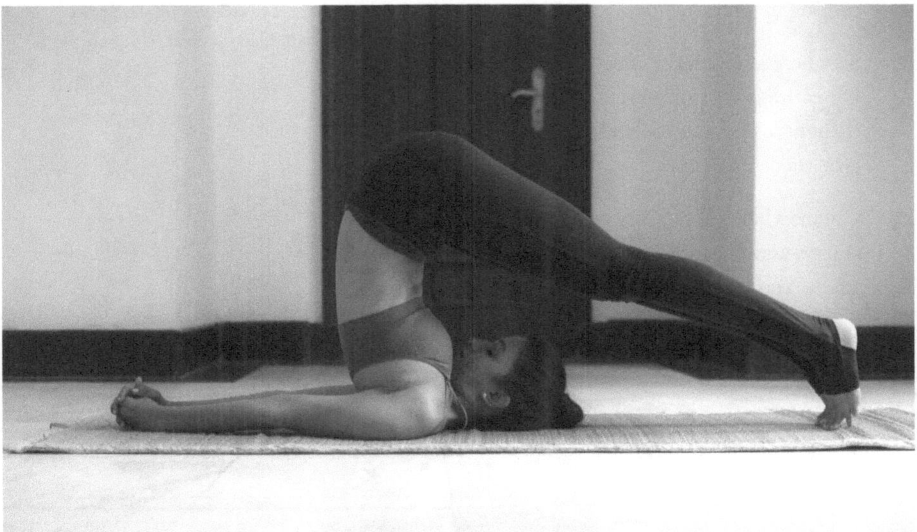

05 – ONE TO THREE MINUTES

urdhva hastasana

UPWARD SALUTE

instructions

1. Stand with the feet together and the arms relaxed by the side
2. Plant both feet firmly on the ground to distribute body weight evenly
3. Raise the arms over the head, interlocking the fingers and turn the palms upward
4. Inhale and stretch the arms up, coming up onto the toes
5. Stay here and breathe, stretching the entire body from top to bottom, without losing balance and remaining grounded
6. On an exhale come down onto the feet and on another inhale, rise on the toes again. You can use this step to re-adjust for balance

benefits

1. Strengthens abdominal muscles
2. Improves alignment and posture

contraindications: Headaches, insomnia, low blood pressure, neck pain/injuries

YOGA TIP:
Keeping your eyes fixed on a focal point in front of you will help you maintain your balance.

your notes:

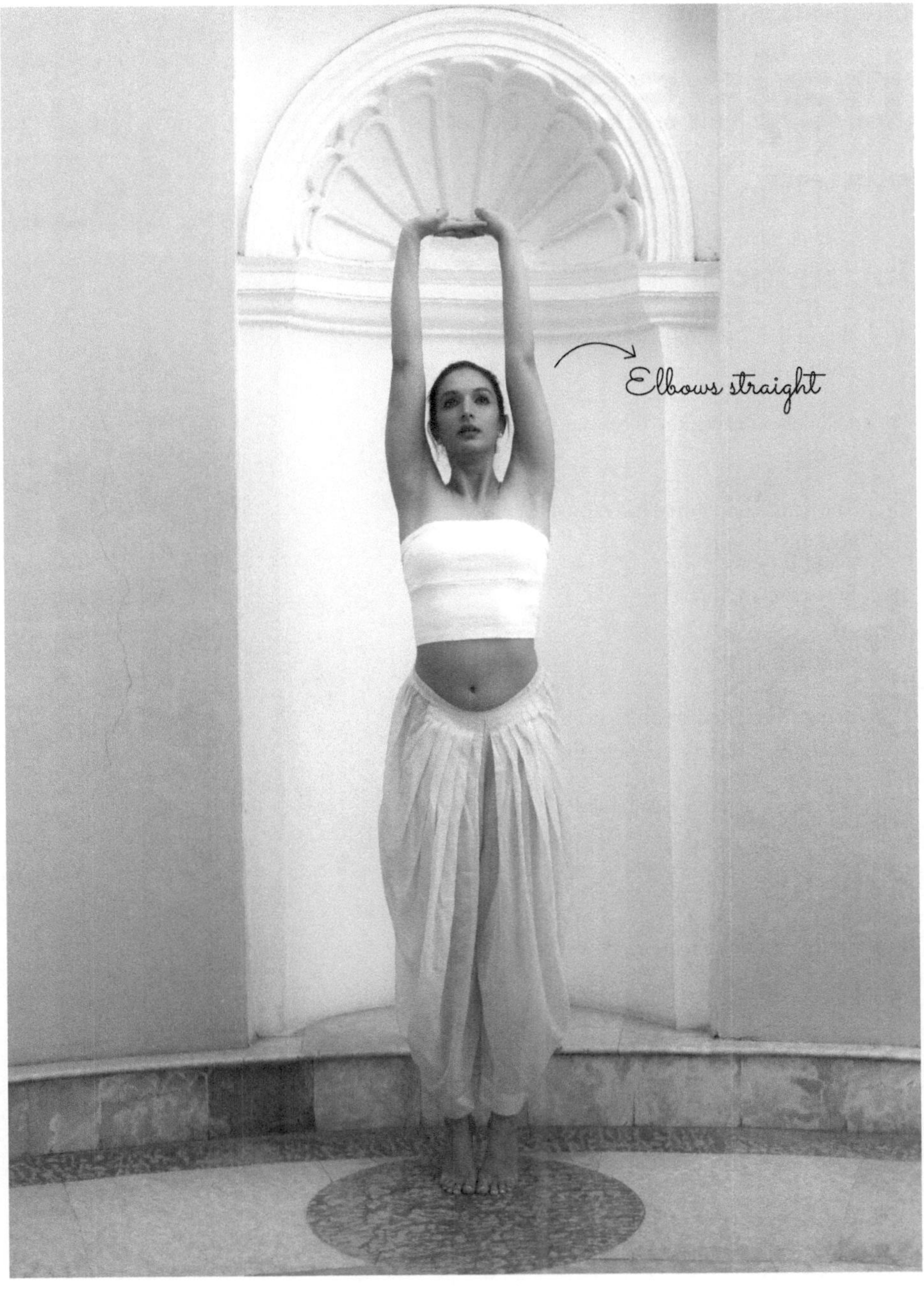
Elbows straight

06 – THIRTY SECONDS

balasana

CHILD'S POSE

instructions

1 Begin in a kneeling pose, sitting on the heels. This is Vajrasana

2 Inhale and bring the forehead on the ground

3 The arms should be placed on either side of the body

4 Stay here and breathe

For an extra stretch:

5 Bring the right arm underneath the left shoulder, look to your right fingers

6 Do the same on the other side

benefits

1 Stretches and relaxes the lower back

2 Stretches the thighs and calf muscles

3 Improves circulation

contraindications: Diarrhoea, pregnancy, knee injuries

your notes:

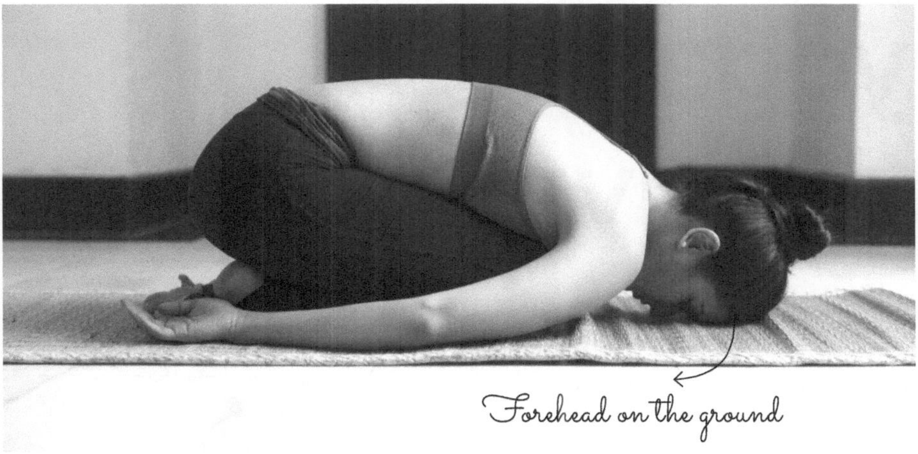

Be gentle with yourself.
You are a child of the
universe. No less than
the trees and the stars.
In the noisy confusion of life
keep the peace in your soul.

- Max Hermann.

yoga for the gym-goer

Some people like workouts which are stimulating, aggressive and that make you sweat. If you're a gym rat, and love pumping iron, yoga may not be your thing. That said, yoga can add to your gym routine even if it doesn't replace it. Gym-goers are typically tight in the hamstrings, quads, chest, and shoulders as a result of traditional strength and cardio training. Yoga can help open these areas up, making them more flexible and less prone to injury so that you can go further in your workout. Incorporating this 10-minute routine into your weekly workout schedule will yield major gains in your flexibility, agility and overall health.

your notes:

01 – TWO MINUTES

anulom vilom

PRANAYAMA

REFER TO PAGE 76

Anulom vilom pranayama helps open your nasal passage so that you can breathe better during your workout and it keeps you focused. It's a great practise to do for 2 minutes before you hit the treadmill.

02 – TWO MINUTES

ardha pincha mayurasana

DOLPHIN POSE

instructions

1. Lower the elbows to the floor placing them directly beneath the shoulders
2. Keep the forearms parallel to each other, distributing the body weight evenly across the forearms
3. Inhale, tuck the toes and lifting the knees off the floor raise the hips toward the ceiling
4. Gaze between the legs
5. Exhale and come down in plank position distributing the weight evenly across the forearms and toes

benefits

1. Stretches the shoulders, hamstrings, calves and arches
2. Strengthens the arms and legs

contraindications: Neck injuries, shoulder injuries

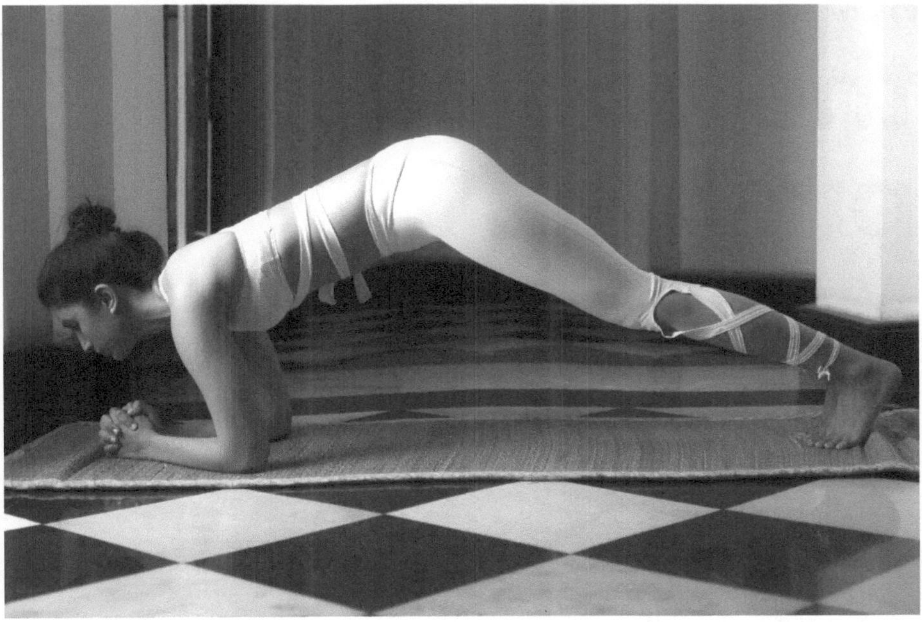

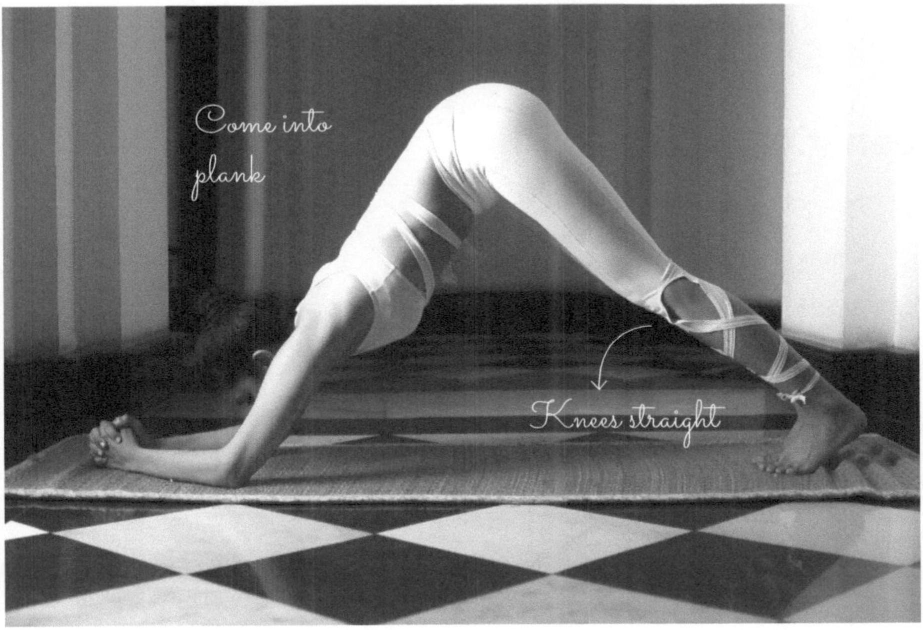

Come into
plank
Knees straight

03 – TWO MINUTES

the yogic push-up

instructions

1. Inhale and bring the body into Downward Dog (Refer to page 106)
2. Exhale lowering the chin and knees to the ground with the hips raised
3. Inhale sliding into Cobra Pose, opening the chest and gazing up toward the ceiling
4. This is one push-up. Continue for two minutes

A great variation on the traditional push-up, the yogic push-up is not only more effective but it also stretches out the shoulders and hamstrings. Do this slowly. The slower you do it, the more effective it is!

benefits

1. Strengthens the arms and back
2. Opens the chest
3. Stretches out the spine, back and chest

your notes:

contraindications: Spinal, knee or back injury

instruction no. 1 on page 106

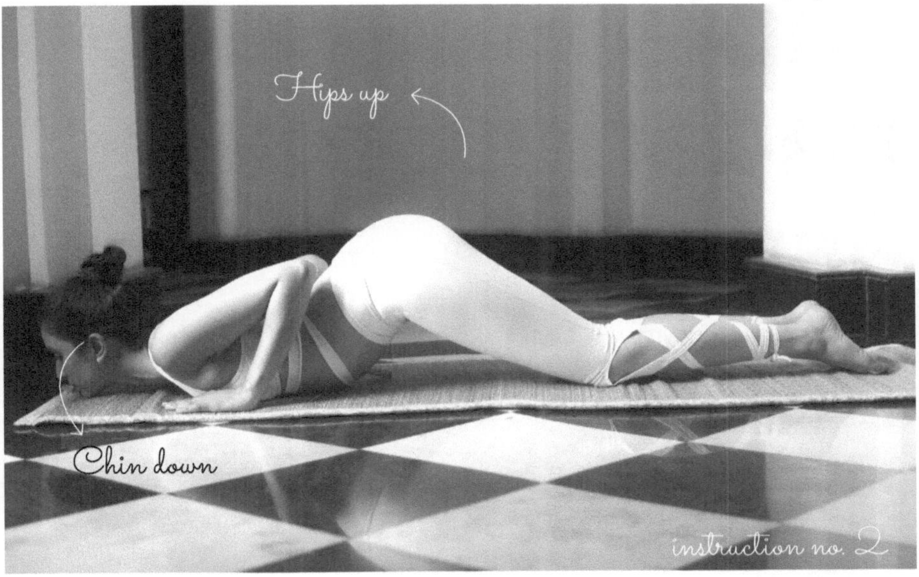

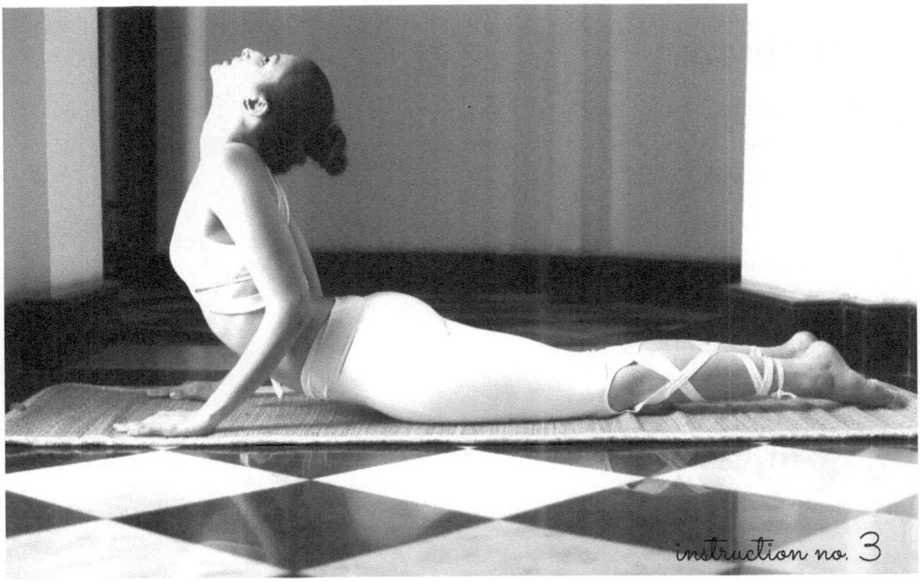

04 – TWO MINUTES

supta padangustha asana

HAMSTRING STRETCH WITH THE BELT

REFER TO PAGE 20

05 – ONE MINUTE

dandasana

STAFF POSE

instructions

1 Sit in a relaxed posture with legs stretched out in front of you. Arms are on the side with palms down on the floor

2 Keeping the spine as straight as possible engage the core and breathe

3 Flex the toes toward the body for an extended stretch

benefits

1 Strengthens the back muscles

2 Lengthens and stretches the spine, shoulder and chest

3 Improves posture

contraindications: Asthma, bronchitis

YOGA TIP:
A simple way to check alignment is to sit with your back against a wall. The shoulder blades should be the only point of contact with the wall.

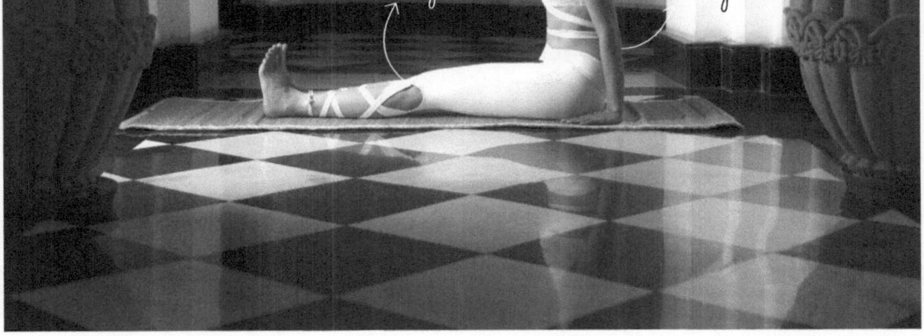

The nature of yoga is to shine the light of awareness into the darkest corners of the body.

– Jason Crandall

06 – ONE MINUTE

shavasana

CORPSE POSE

REFER TO PAGE 28

yoga for lazy people

Lots of people tell me that while they want to practise yoga, they are just too lazy and can't seem to get off the couch. Well, no worries. Yoga can be done by the laziest of the laziest. And the good news is – you don't even have to get off your couch. Just stay where you are and do this routine; I guarantee that you will be abuzz with positive energy afterwards. Though easy and simple to do, these pranayama and asanas have profound health and mental benefits, and can be the easiest solution to drive that lethargy away.

your notes:

01 – TWO MINUTES

surya bheda

PRANAYAMA

instructions

1. Sit up straight in a comfortable, relaxed posture
2. Close the eyes. On the right hand, bend the index and middle fingers applying Vishnu mudra and bring the thumb and forefinger to Gyan mudra on the left
3. Inhale through the right nostril, retain the breath for a moment and exhale through the left
4. Repeat, inhaling through the right nostril and exhaling through the left

This pranayama is called the Surya Bheda as it stimulates the solar or pingala nadi of the body, which is influenced by the sun.

YOGA TIP:
Always allow for an interval of at least 3 hours before or after eating when you do this pranayama as it produces a lot of heat in the body.

Your body is made up of three gunas: sattva *(peace and calm),* rajas *(activity) and* tamas *(inertia). When you are lazy, tamas has increased. The aim of doing these practices is to drive tamas away.*

benefits

1. Energizing
2. Detoxifies the blood
3. Improves digestion
4. Alleviates symptoms of ageing

contraindications: High blood pressure

your notes:

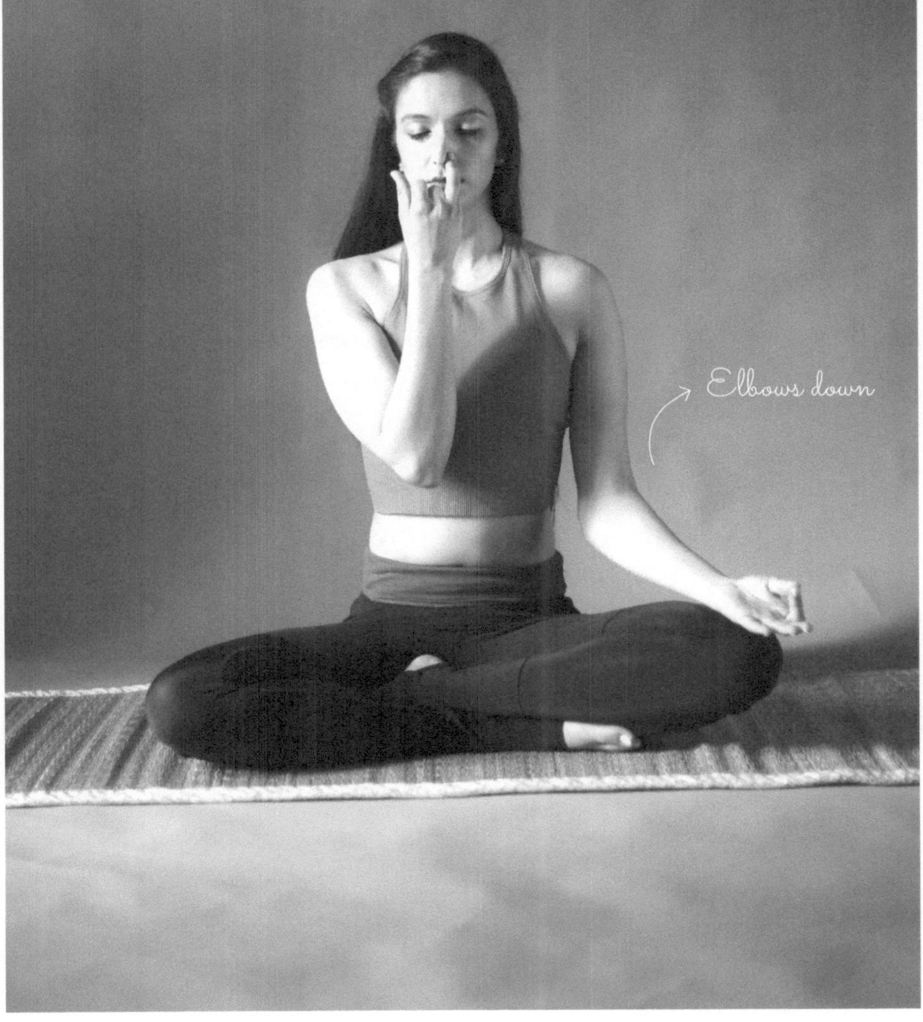
Elbows down

02 – TWO MINUTES

dolasana

PENDULUM POSE

instructions

1. Stand up straight with the left and right foot 2 feet apart and the arms on either side of the body
2. Inhale, raising the arms, clasping them just above the head
3. Exhale and bend over at the waist
4. Retain the breath as you swing from side to side, with the forehead tapping one knee and then the other
5. Exhale and return to a standing position. Repeat a few more times

benefits

1. Stretches the hamstrings
2. Strengthens the spine and stimulates the central nervous system
3. Improves circulation to the head and face

contraindications: Heart disease, high blood pressure

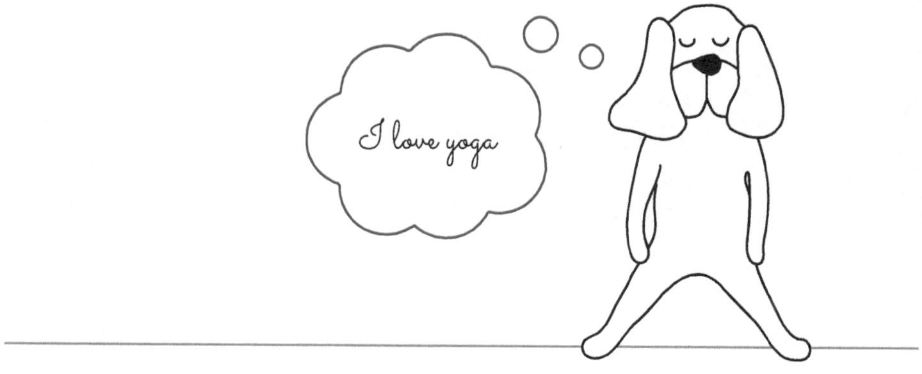

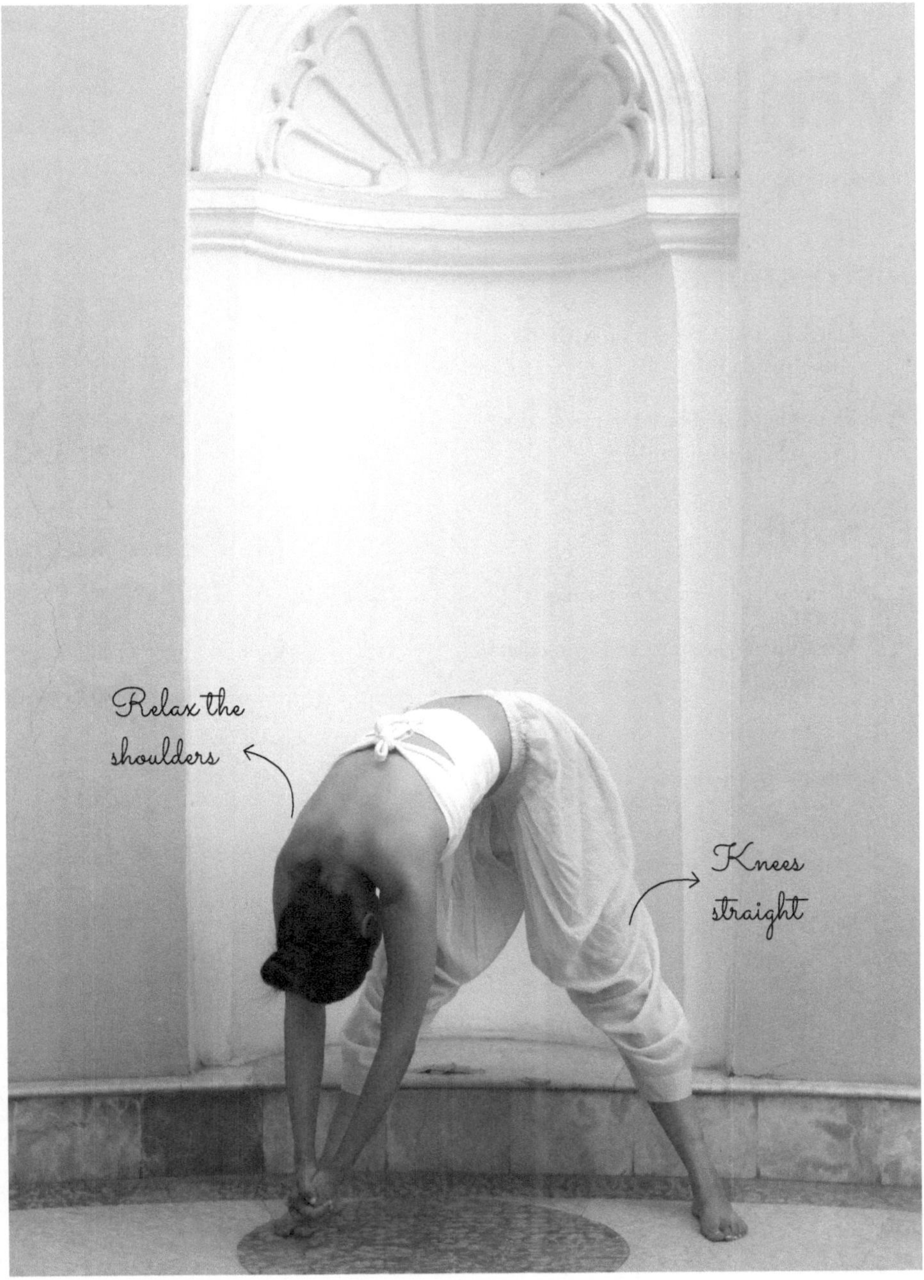
Relax the shoulders
Knees straight

03 – TWO MINUTES

vajrasana

DIAMOND POSE

instructions

1 Come in a seated position with the legs under the body

2 The spine should be straight and the knees close to each other

benefits

1 Stretches the muscles of the legs

2 Strengthens the spine and stimulates the central nervous system

your notes:

contraindications: Knee injuries

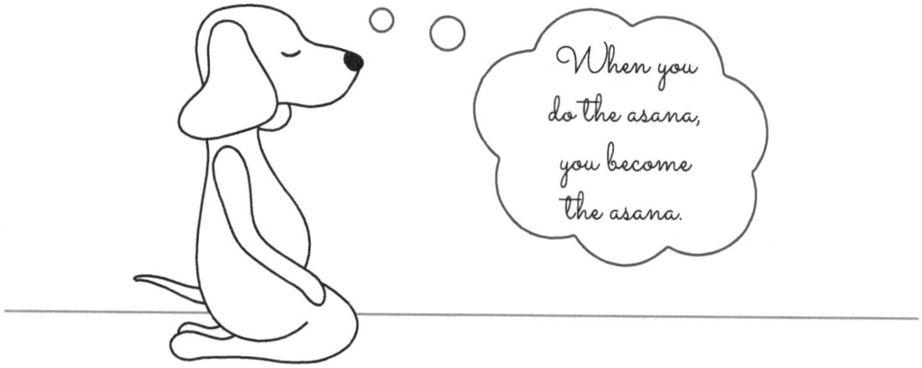

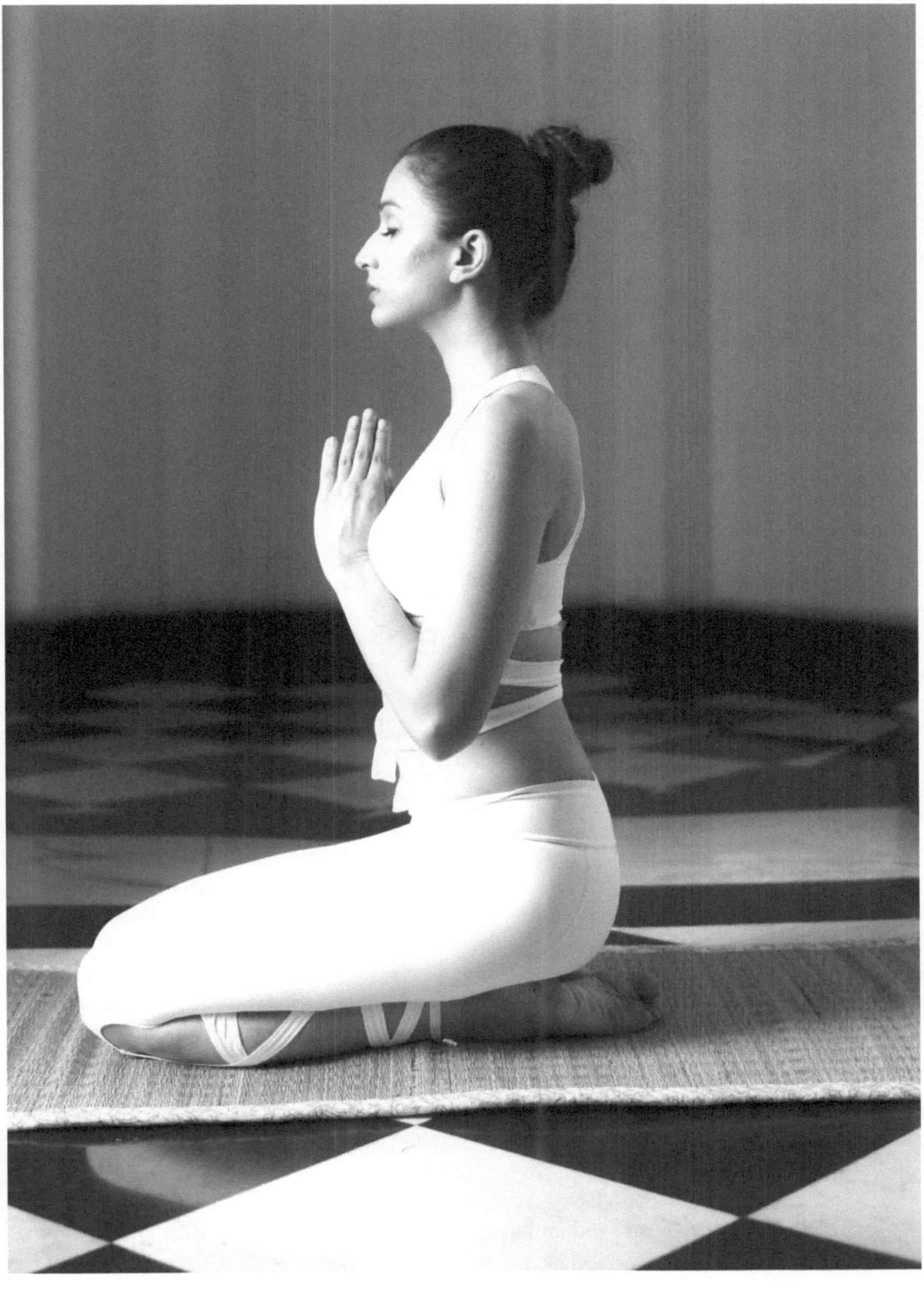

04 – TWO MINUTES

padmasana / ardha padmasana

LOTUS POSE
IRA'S FAVOURITE ASANA

instructions

1. Sit up straight in a comfortable, relaxed posture with the legs extended in front of you
2. Bend the right knee placing the right foot on the left thigh. The sole of the foot should be turned upward and the heel close to the abdomen
3. Repeat on the left side
4. With both legs crossed bring the thumb to forefinger in Gyan mudra
5. Close the eyes and breathe mindfully, remaining here for a few minutes

benefits

1. Calms the brain
2. Stimulates the pelvic and abdominal areas, as well as the spine and bladder
3. Stretches the ankles and knees
4. Alleviates menstrual discomfort
5. Relieves sciatic pain

contraindications: Knee injuries, ankle injuries

YOGA FACT:
Yoga master B.K.S. Iyengar believed that the Padmasana is the only pose in which all four areas of the body are perfectly balanced: the feet, legs, and pelvis; the torso; the arms and hands; and the neck, throat, and head. When the body achieves perfect balance, Iyengar says, the brain can rest correctly on the spinal column and breathing comes easily.

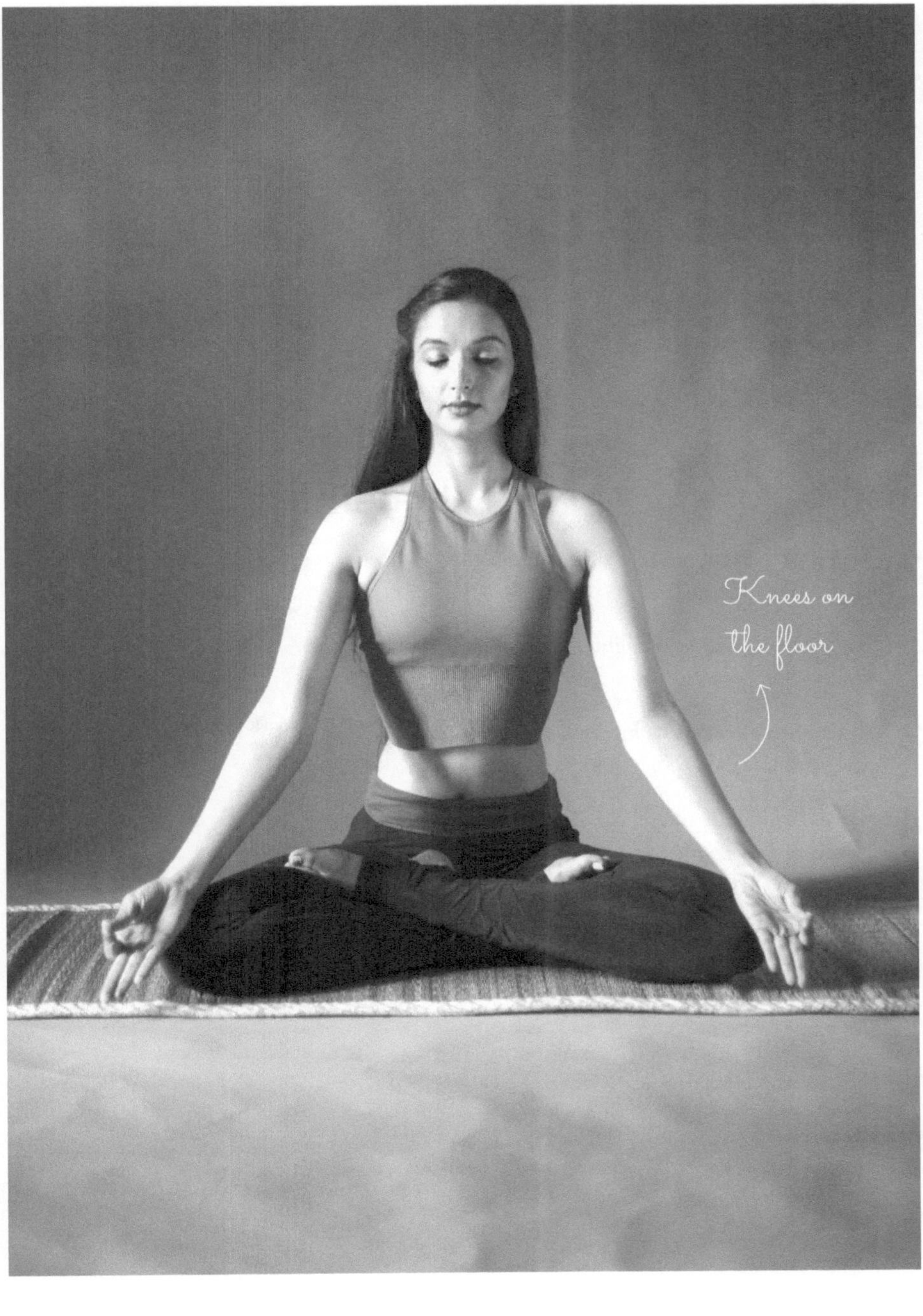
Knees on
the floor

05 – TWO MINUTES

simha garjana asana

ROARING LION POSE

instructions

1. Kneel in a seated position with the legs under the body
2. The spine should be straight and the knees slightly apart
3. Place the palms on the knees, keeping the arms relaxed
4. Open the mouth and relax the jaw, allowing the tongue to hang loosely
5. Breathe through the nose and mouth
6. Engaging the core and contracting the abdominal muscles retain the breath for a few seconds
7. Exhale and relax
8. Repeat for a few rounds

benefits

1. Relieves tension in the chest and face
2. Stabilizes the body and eradicates disease

contraindications: Knee injuries

your notes:

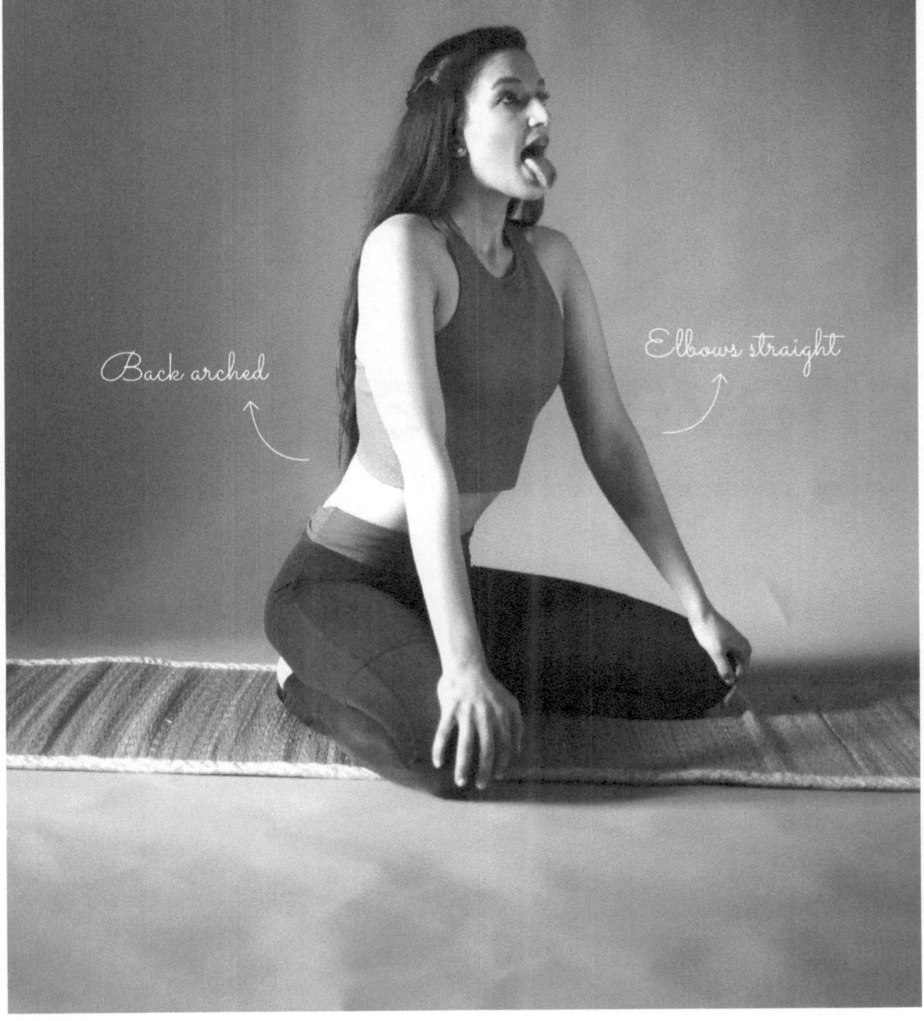
Back arched
Elbows straight

06 – ONE MINUTE

sarpasana

SNAKE POSE

REFER TO PAGE 24

your notes:

07 – ONE MINUTE

shavasana

THIS IS A LAZY PERSON'S FAVOURITE ASANA!

REFER TO PAGE 28

your notes:

yoga to tone hips and thighs

Big hips and jiggly thighs can be a problem for most people. These two body parts are most susceptible to weight gain, and are also areas where weight loss is more difficult. Yoga can not only help slim and tone these areas through targeted practise, but can also help open the hips, pelvis and hamstring muscles to prevent injury and stiffness. This 10-minute routine is particularly helpful for women for whom the hip-thigh area can often be a 'danger zone'. After all, everyone wants to be able to fit into their skinny jeans.

your notes:

01 – TWO MINUTES

vyaghrasana

TIGER POSE

instructions

1. Begin by coming onto all fours, your palms and knees on the ground
2. Inhale, arch the back, drop the abdomen and raise the right leg and chin towards the sky
3. Stay here for a few seconds and retain the breath
4. Exhale, arch the back upwards bringing the right knee and chin towards the chest
5. Repeat on the other side

benefits

1. Stimulates weight loss in the hips and thighs
2. Relieves tension in the back
3. Stimulates the spinal nerves
4. Improves digestion

contraindications: Knee injuries, back injuries

Yoga does not just change the way we see things, it transforms the person who sees.

– BKS Iyengar

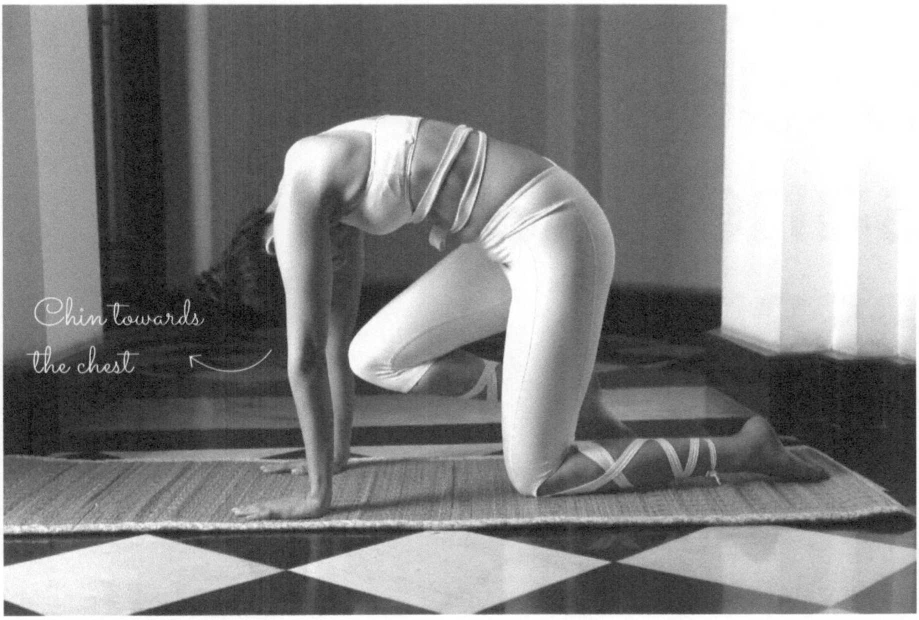
Chin towards
the chest

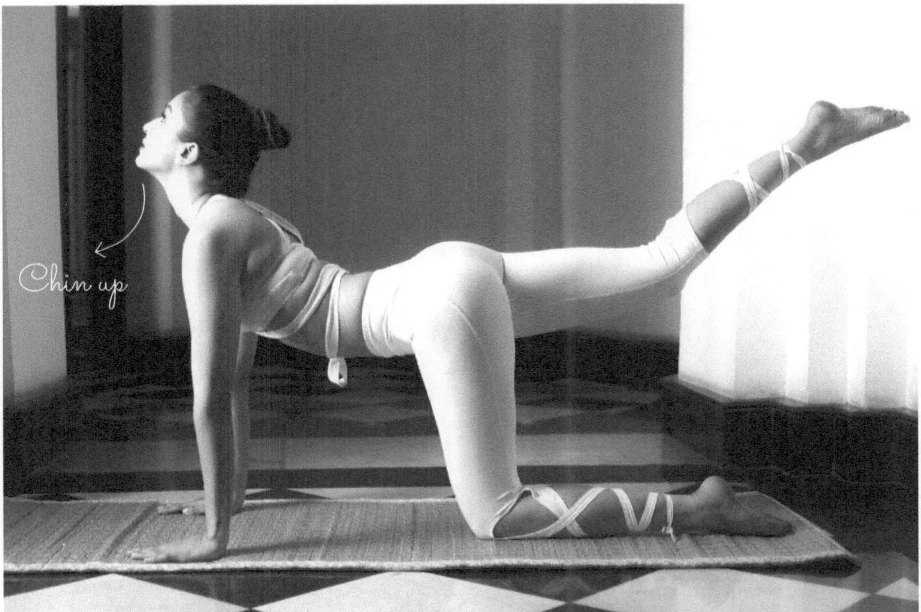
Chin up

02 – TWO MINUTES

pada sanchalan asana

YOGIC CYCLING

instructions

1 Lie flat on the back with arms on either side of the body

2 Bring the right leg up, pulling the knee towards the chest, and practise a cycling movement

3 Inhale as you straighten the leg, and exhale as you bend the knee

4 Practice this for a minute and then switch directions. If you begin clockwise then switch to anti-clockwise and vice versa

benefits

1 Strengthens the pelvic and knee joints

2 Strengthens abdominal and back muscles

3 Tones the thighs and waist

contraindications: High blood pressure, heart disease, menstruation, pregnancy, hernia, abdominal surgery

YOGA TIP:
If you find this difficult, place the arms underneath your body. Place the arms behind the head for an extra challenge.

your notes:

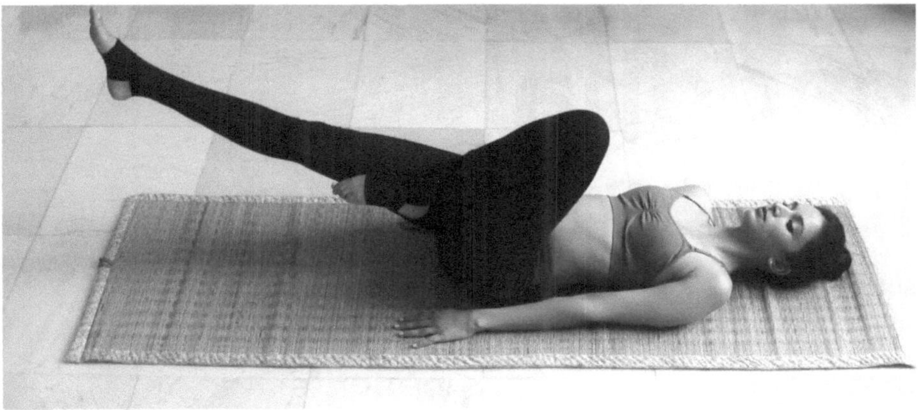

Never underestimate
a woman with a yoga mat!

your notes:

03 – TWO MINUTES

baddha konasana

BUTTERFLY POSE

instructions

1. Sit up with the legs extended in front of you
2. Bending both knees, bring the soles of both feet together and grab the big toes
3. Keeping the back straight, flap the thighs up and down to mimic a butterfly's wings
4. As you inhale and exhale, you should be able to pull the feet closer toward the body and relax deeper into the pose

benefits

1. Stretches the spine and back
2. Relaxes the pelvic muscles

contraindications: Pelvic surgery or injuries, knee injuries

your notes:

---

04 – TWO MINUTES

anjaneya asana

CRESCENT MOON POSE

REFER TO PAGE 108

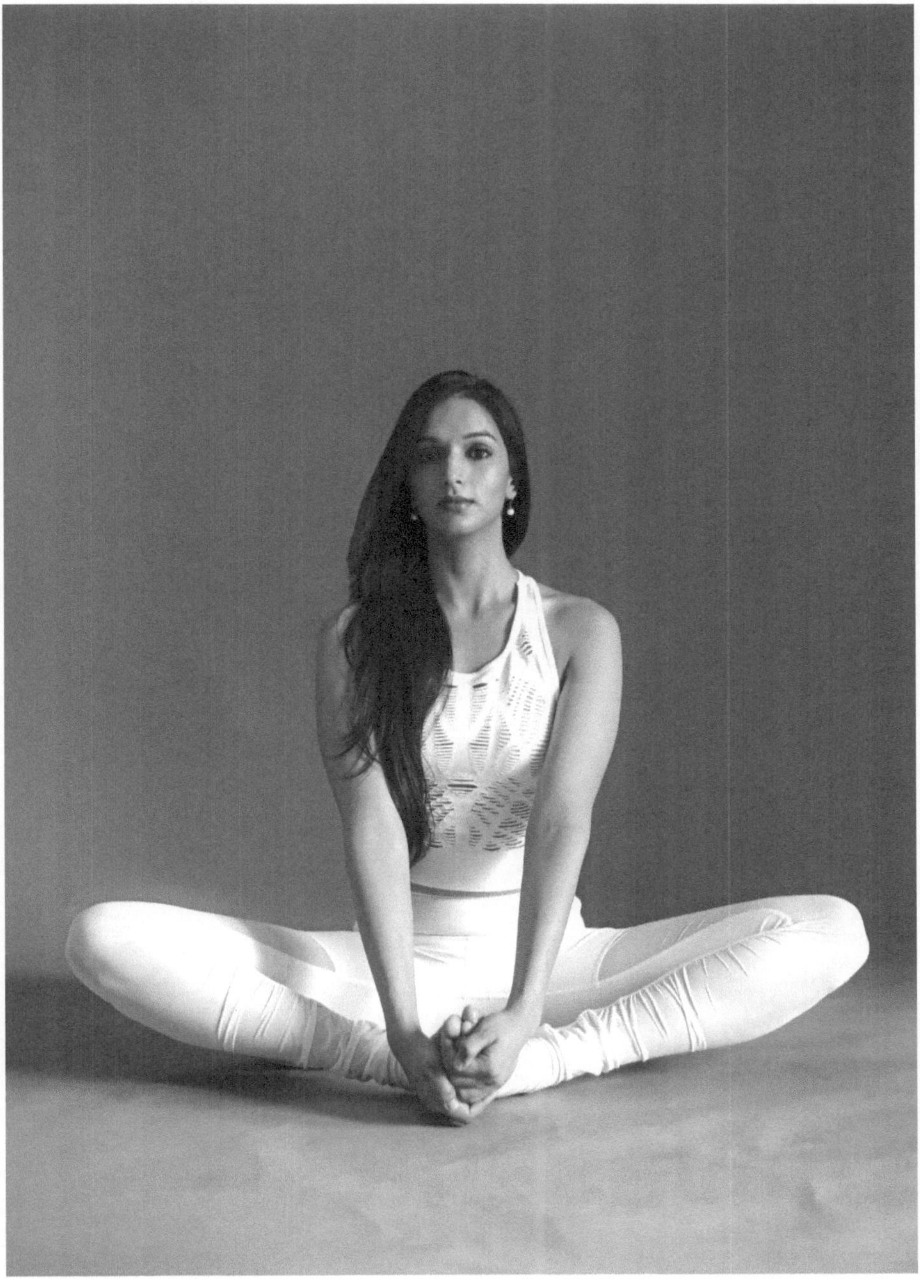

05 – TWO MINUTES

trikonasana

TRIANGLE POSE

instructions

1. Stand up on the mat with the left and right foot 3-4 feet apart
2. Extend the arms straight out on either side comfortably at shoulder level so as not to strain the neck or shoulders
3. Inhale, turn the right foot to a 90-degree angle, exhale, placing the right hand on the knee, shin or ankle
4. The left arm should be extended towards the ceiling. Gaze towards the left hand
5. Stay here and breathe focusing on the stretch the thighs and hips
6. Exhale and straighten the right leg, bringing the arms back to shoulder level
7. Repeat on the left side

benefits

1. Strengthens and stretches the hips
2. Stretches the pelvic muscles improving flexibility
3. Tones the inner thighs
4. Strengthens the spine

contraindications: Spinal disc herniation, back pain or injuries

your notes:

---

06 – THIRTY SECONDS

shavasana

CORPSE POSE

REFER TO PAGE 28

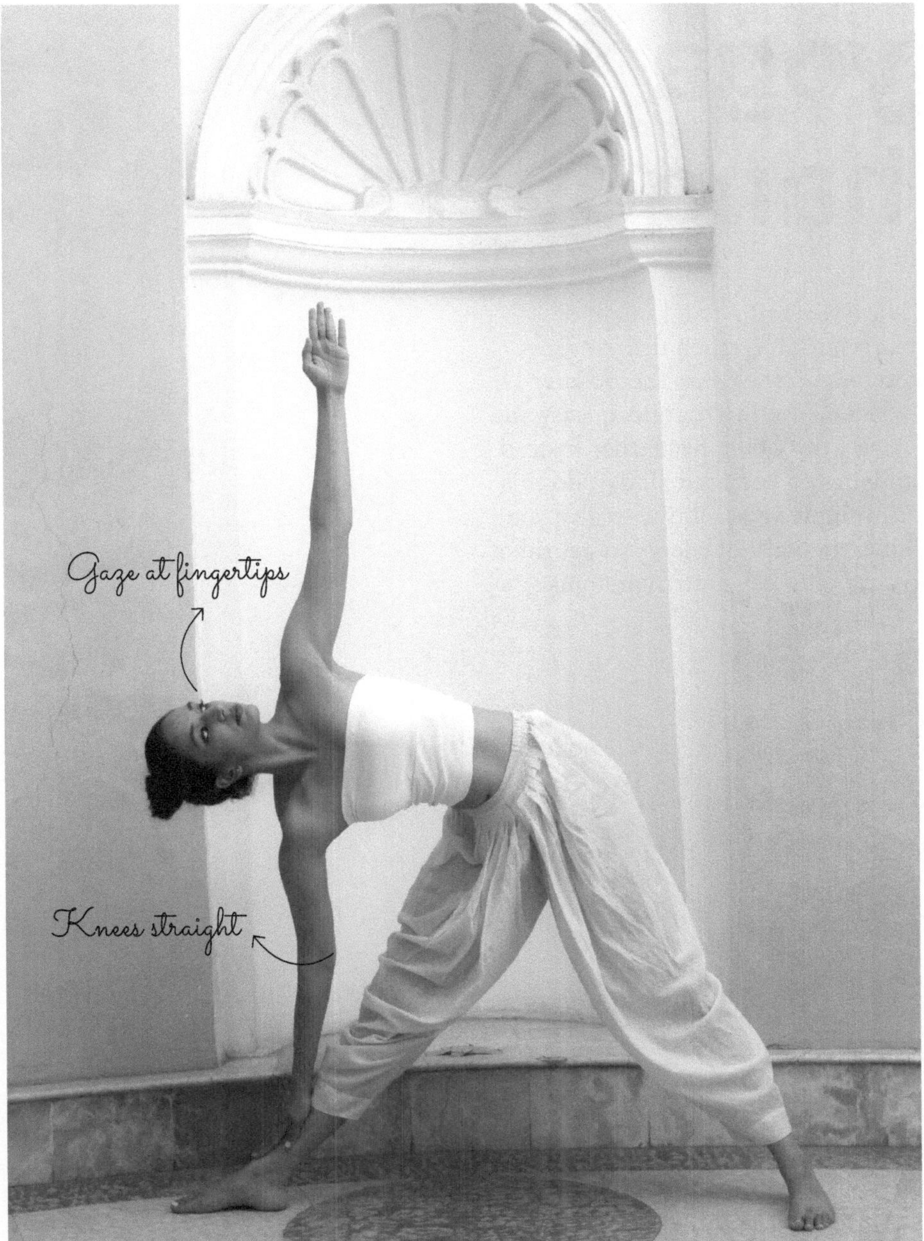
Gaze at fingertips
Knees straight

yoga for hangovers

Have you had a rough night of partying? Too much drinking? Smoking? Stayed up far too late? Do you feel utterly lethargic, queasy and have a throbbing headache? Instead of lying on your bed all day, do this 10-minute yoga routine to give you an extra boost of energy to get rid of your pesky hangover symptoms.

your notes:

01 – TWO MINUTES

kapalabhati

REFER TO PAGE 16

This kriya balances the nervous system, energizes the mind and body, removes grogginess and allows the body to take in copious amounts of oxygen, which is vital if you have a bad hangover. Begin with 2 minutes of this practise, but try to increase it to 6-7 minutes if you have a particularly bad hangover.

instructions

Add breath retention to the standard Kapalabhati practise for additional oxygenation.

1. After one round of 20 pumpings, take a deep breath in and retain the breath for 20-30 seconds
2. Begin the next round
3. Add a retention

benefits

1. Improves oxygenation to the body
2. Calms and focuses the mind
3. Alleviates symptoms of drinking (like headaches) through detoxification

contraindications: Asthma, respiratory diseases

your notes:

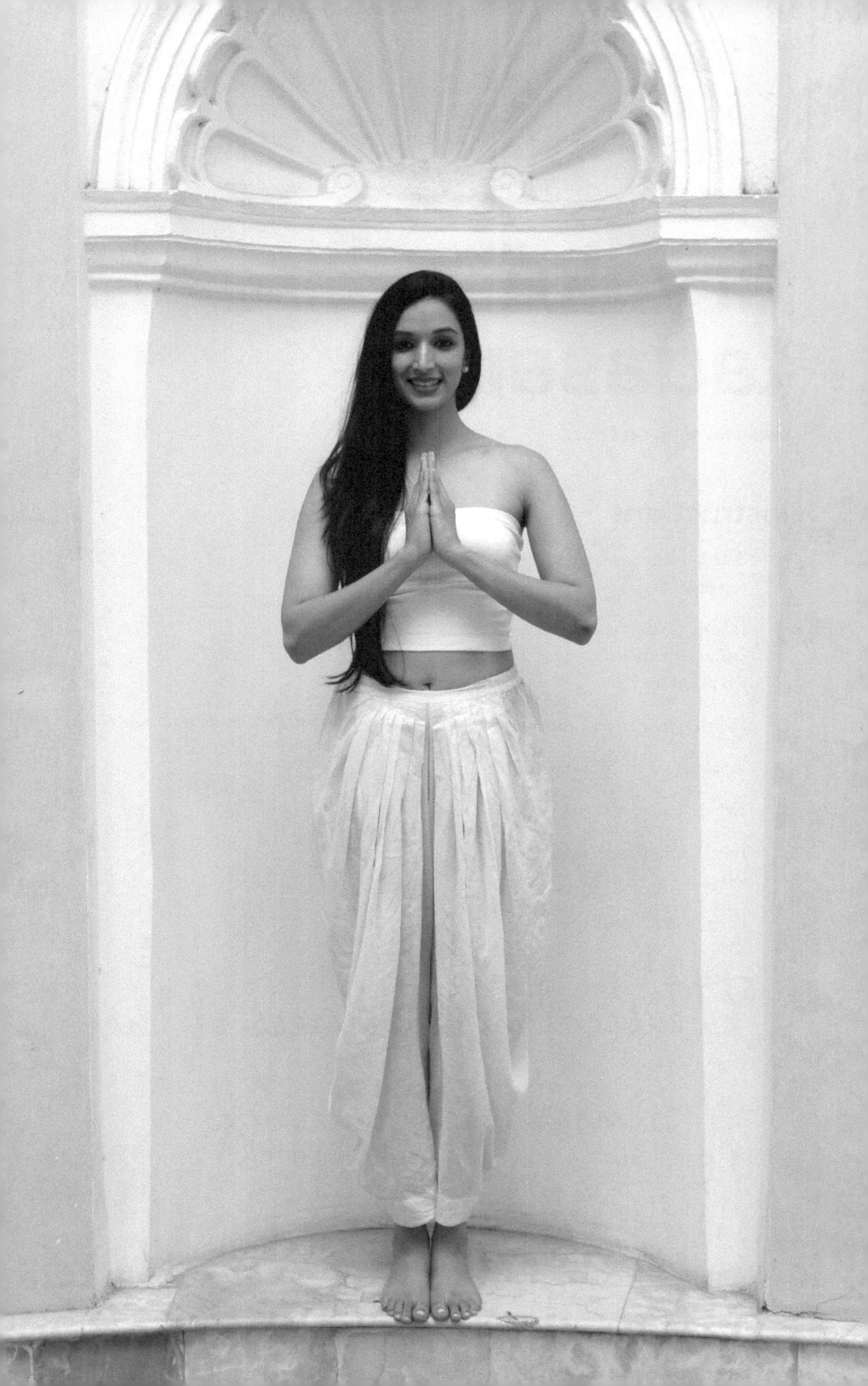

02 – TWO MINUTES

tiryaka tadasana

SWINGING PALM TREE POSE

instructions

1 Stand up on the mat with the feet 3-4 feet apart

2 Inhale, raising the arms up toward the ceiling, interlace the fingers and turn the palms up

3 Exhale, straightening the spine

4 Inhale, bend the arms toward the right

5 Exhale, return to centre

6 Inhale, bending the arms toward the left

7 Exhale, return to centre

benefits

1 Relaxes the body and mind

2 Improves blood circulation

3 Balances the nervous system

contraindications: Neck injuries, headaches, low blood pressure, pregnancy

This calm steadiness of the senses is called yoga.

– Katha Upanishad

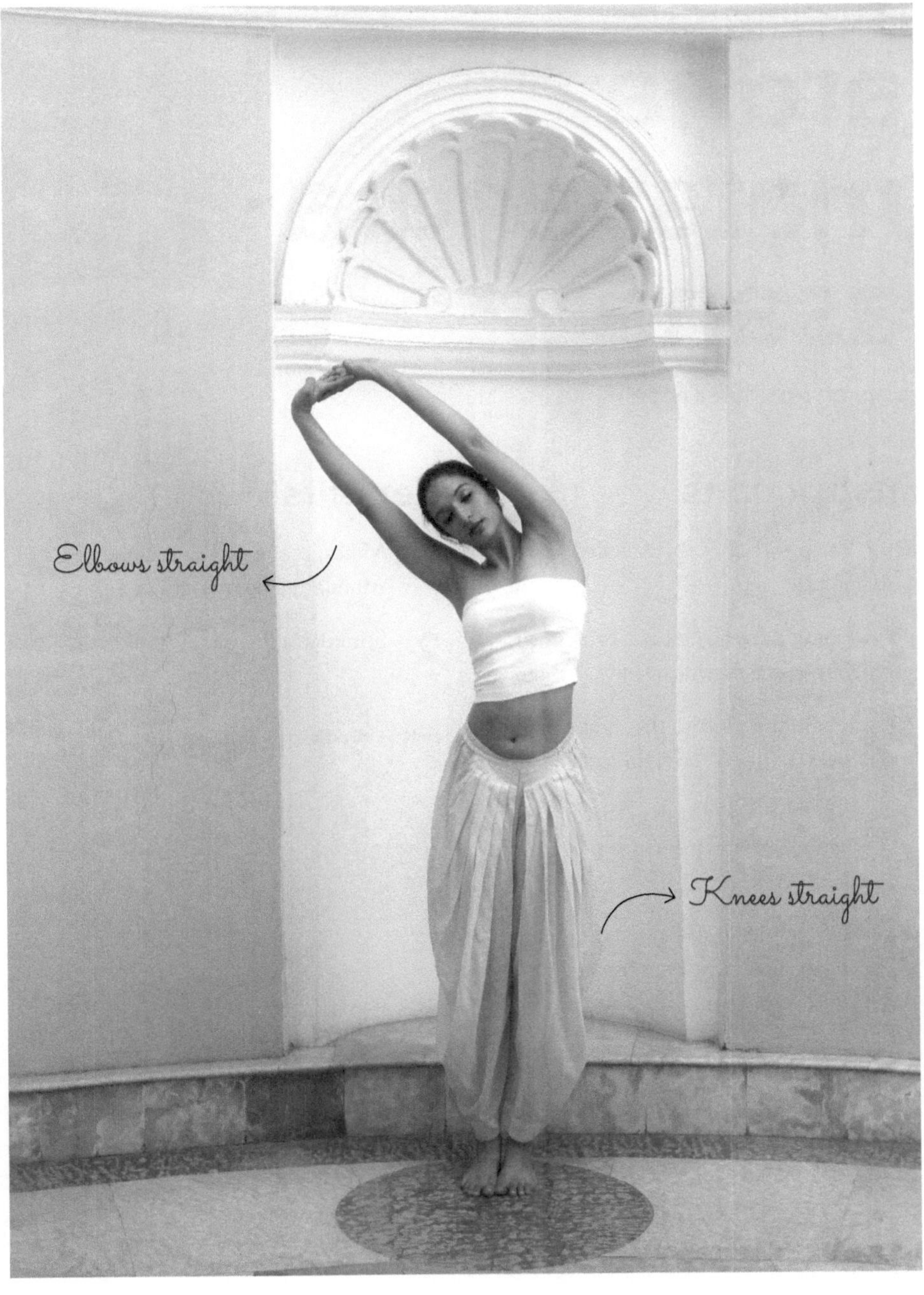
Elbows straight
Knees straight

03 – TWO MINUTES

ardha matsyendra asana

LORD OF THE FISHES POSE

instructions

1. Sit up with the legs extended in front of you
2. Bending the right knee, bring the right foot on the outside of the left thigh
3. Inhale and twist to the right bringing the left arm by the right leg
4. Place the right hand on the floor behind you and gaze over the right shoulder
5. As you inhale, straighten the spine, and exhale, twist even further
6. Repeat on the other side

benefits

1. Massages the liver and kidneys stimulating detoxification
2. Stimulates the spinal cord

contraindications: Back injuries, spinal injuries

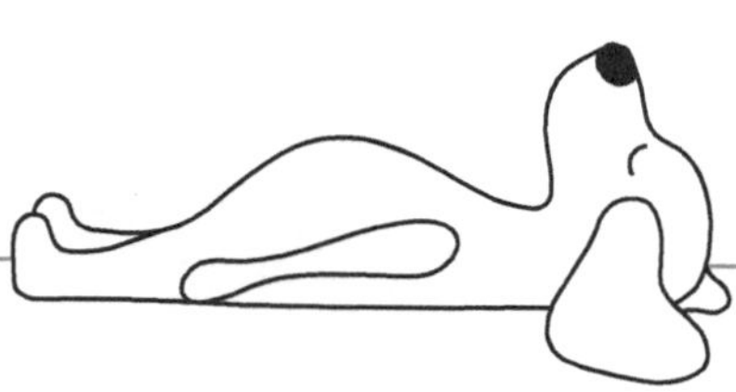

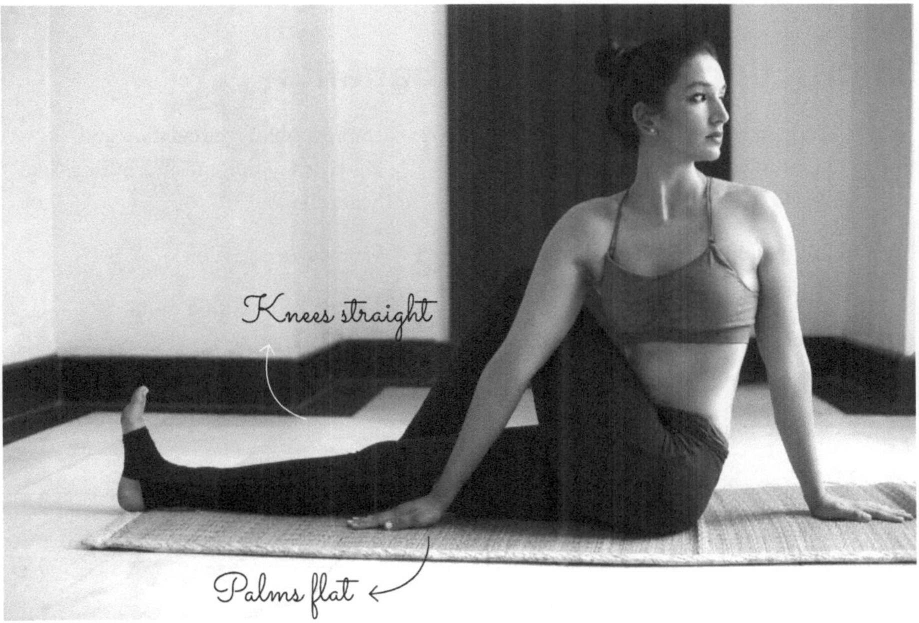
Knees straight
Palms flat

04 – ONE AND A HALF MINUTES

sethu bandhasana

BRIDGE POSE

instructions

1. Laying on your back with arms on your side, bend your knees bringing the feet closer to the body
2. Raise the hips up keeping the feet fixed on the ground
3. Support your lower back with your palms
4. Stay here and breathe
5. If you can't hold this posture, do this as a dynamic exercise and then hold as long as you can

benefits

1. Improves blood circulation and alleviates symptoms of drinking (like headaches)
2. Stimulates digestion
3. Calms the body and mind
4. Rejuvenates the body

contraindications: Neck injuries, back injuries, wrist injuries

your notes:

05 – ONE AND A HALF MINUTES

sasang asana

REFER TO PAGE 34

your notes:

06 – ONE MINUTE

shavasana

REFER TO PAGE 28

The journey of a million miles begins with a single step

- Lao Tzu

yoga to quit smoking

Smoking is a terrible habit; everyone knows this. But it's also a *terribly* difficult habit to kick. Yoga can help you effectively quit smoking by working on your pranic energy and purifying the *nadis* in your body. Yoga creates a subconscious sense of control which will help you conquer strong tobacco cravings and the urge to smoke. It's a slow process but a solid and long-term solution to a damaging habit. Yoga can also help you deal with some of the side-effects of smoking by strengthening your lungs and detoxifying the body.

your notes:

01 – TWO MINUTES

dolasana

PENDULUM POSE

REFER TO PAGE 132

benefits

1. Improves breathing capacity
2. Improves blood circulation
3. Warms up the body
4. Relieves tension in the neck, back and shoulders

contraindications: Severe back pain, heart disease, high blood pressure

YOGA TIP:
This dynamic asana looks easy but it has numerous benefits if done with focus and proper breathing.

02 – TWO MINUTES

kundalini breath

instructions

1. Sit up straight in a comfortable, relaxed posture
2. Resting both hands on the knees, bring together the thumb and forefinger in Gyan mudra
3. Inhale deeply from the tummy, lifting the chest up
4. Exhale, twist to the right and gaze over the right shoulder
5. Return to centre. Repeat on the other side
6. Continue for 2 minutes remaining mindful of the breath

benefits

1 Increased oxygenation

2 Detoxifies the body

3 Purifies the respiratory system

4 Improves blood circulation

> **YOGA TIP:**
> Pranayama is the main force behind mind control. By practising pranayama, you are subconsciously activating cues to your mind and body that you are in total control of your actions.

contraindications: Vertigo

03 – TWO MINUTES

anulom vilom

ALTERNATE NOSTRIL BREATHING WITH COUNTING

REFER TO PAGE 76

benefits

1 Purifies the respiratory system

2 Increases circulation

3 Profound calming and relaxing effect on the body, mind and pranic system

> **YOGA TIP:**
> The longer you do this practise the better. Increasing your time from 2 minutes to 5 minutes is a good idea, especially if you are very hungover.

contraindications: None!

your notes:

04 – TWO MINUTES

ashwa sanchalan asana

EQUESTRIAN POSE

instructions

1. Begin by coming on to all fours
2. Extend the left leg out toward the back
3. Step the right foot between the two hands and open the chest with the shoulders back
4. Tilt the chin upward, gazing toward the ceiling, your arms by your side
5. Breathe and sink the hips toward the ground, relaxing deeper into the pose
6. Repeat on the other side

benefits

1. Stretches the spine
2. Massages the internal organs detoxifying the body
3. Alleviates tension in the chest and shoulders

contraindications: Knee injuries, back injuries

your notes:

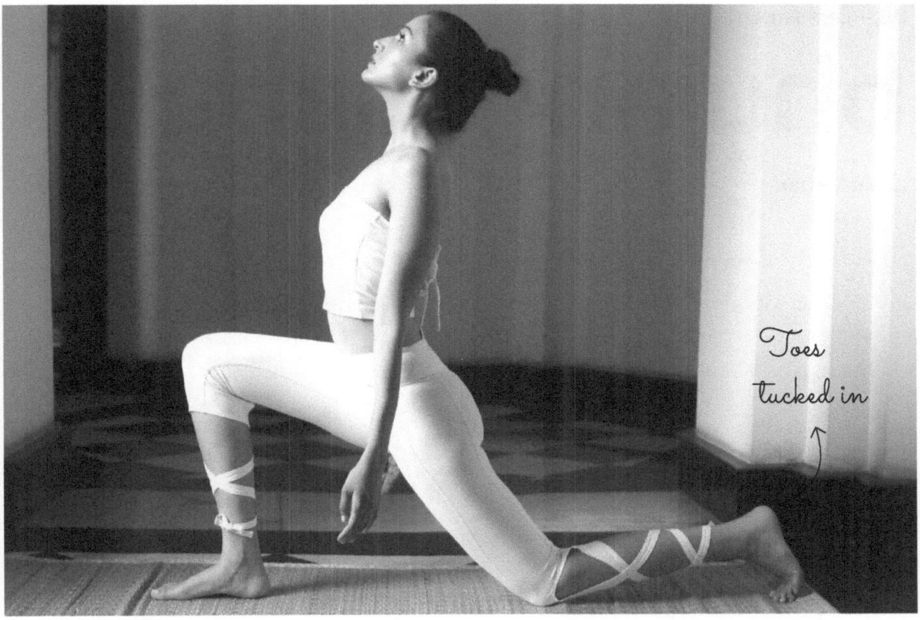

For a yogi nothing is impossible.

– Swami Vishnudevananda.

05 – ONE MINUTE

bhujangasana

COBRA POSE

REFER TO PAGE 80

This asana will get your digestion up and running, and will get rid of the uncomfortable bloating that comes with a hangover.

your notes:

06 – ONE MINUTE

balasana

CHILD'S POSE

REFER TO PAGE 118

your notes:

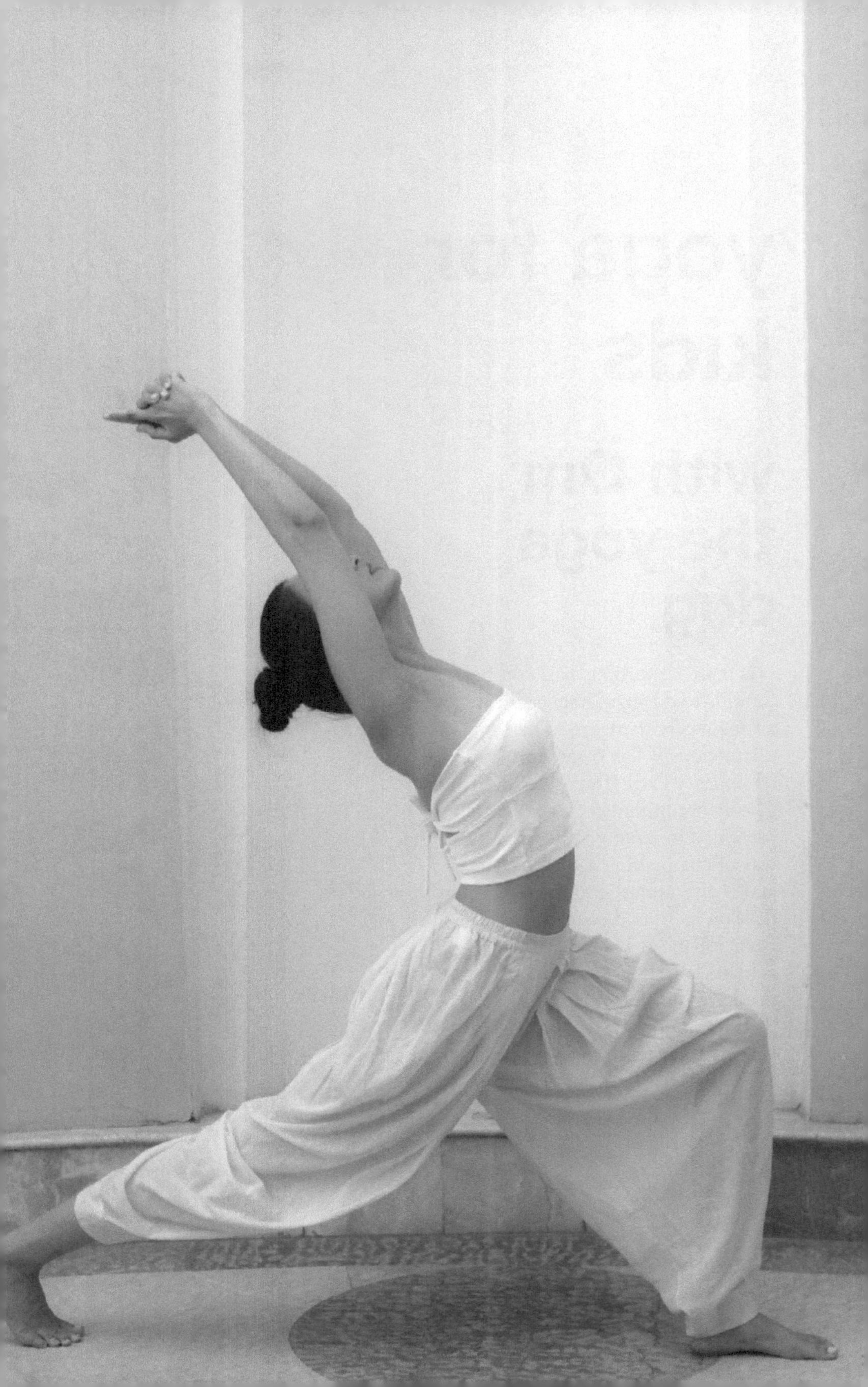

yoga for kids

with Om the yoga dog

It is more important than ever before for kids to do yoga. Especially at a time where there are so many distractions – TV, computers, i-Phones, i-Pads. Today, children are grossly overstimulated. Yoga, when presented in a fun way, is a great way of channelling a child's energy and is also fantastic for helping them develop focus and concentration. Remember, seeds sown early reap benefits later in life. In this chapter, you have Om the Yoga Dog, Prana the Frog and Moksha Elephant sharing their teachings with kids.

your notes:

01 – TWO MINUTES

heart and belly breath

instructions

1 Sit in a comfortable position with your spine straight. Place one hand on your tummy and another one on your chest. Close your eyes. Notice how your breath is moving in and out of your body

2 Inhale and exhale paying attention to your breath. Inhale and let your tummy get big by filling it with your breath. As you exhale, pull your belly button in, pushing all the air out

3 Breathe like this, focussing on your breath, breathing slowly and comfortably

4 Breathe deeply. Imagine that you are breathing into your heart. Fill your tummy with air. Breathe a little bit more bringing the breath to your chest

5 Exhale. Squeeze the air out of your heart and then your tummy

6 Continue this breathing – filling your tummy with air, then your heart and then exhaling from your heart and your tummy

benefits

1 Oxygenates the body

2 Builds focus

3 Calms the mind

contraindications: None!

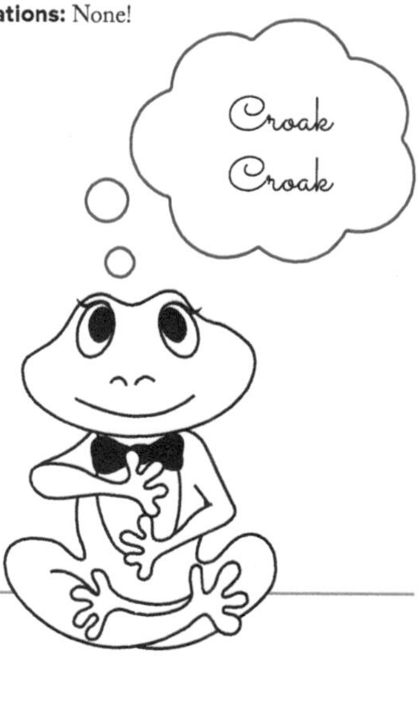

02 – TWO MINUTES

cycling

instructions

1 Lie down on your back on the mat, arms by your side, raise both legs off the mat and imagine that you are cycling. Breathe steadily, inhaling and exhaling

2 Continue this for a minute. Now reverse the direction of cycling

benefits

1 Great way to spend that extra energy

2 Good for digestion

3 Lots of fun to do

contraindications: Severe neck, spine or back problems

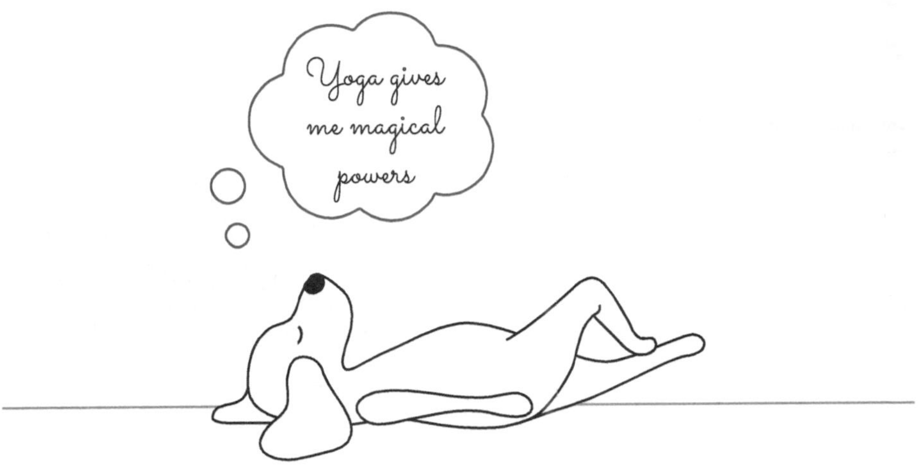

03 – TWO MINUTES

bridge

instructions

1 Lie down with your back on the mat. Bring your arms by your side

2 Bend your knees and bring your heels close to the buttocks. Your feet should be a foot apart

3 Slowly raise your stomach, supporting your lower back with your hands

4 Hold this position for a few seconds and breathe. Gently come down

YOGA FACT:
This asana is difficult for adults to do but is easy enough for kids, who are naturally more flexible.

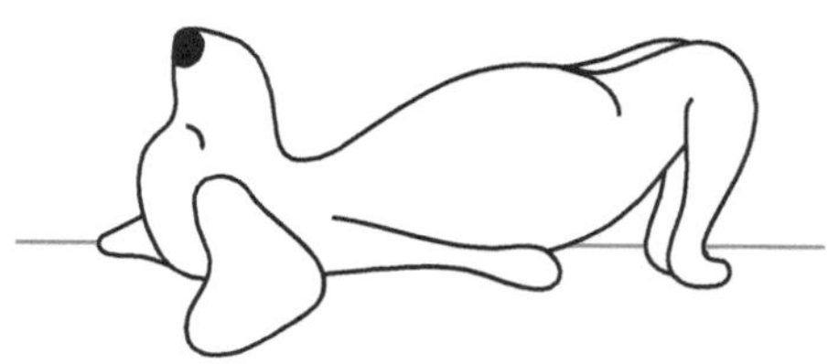

benefits

1 Builds confidence

2 Improves flexibility

3 Gets rid of fear

contraindications: Severe neck, spine or back problems

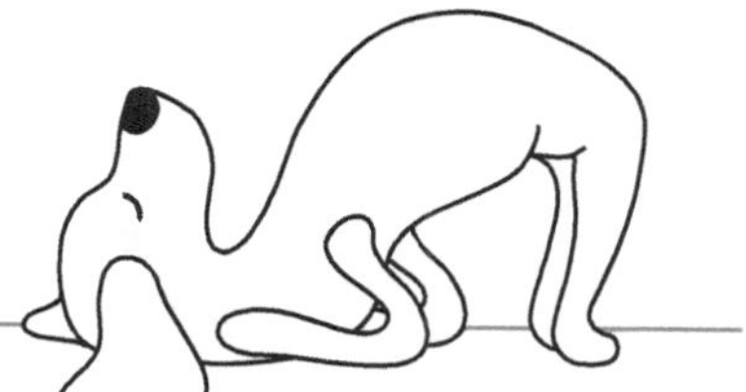

04 – TWO MINUTES

butterfly

instructions

1 Sit with your legs straight out in front of you. Bend your knees and pull your heels towards your pelvis

2 Drop your knees out to the sides and press the soles of your feet together, bringing your heels as close to the pelvis as you can

3 Hold your toes. Inhale and exhale with control. Flap your knees up and down like a butterfly

benefits

1 Great for hips and knees (prevents serious injuries from all those falls)

2 Teaches kids to sit still

3 Reduces stress and anxiety

contraindications: Serious hip or knee problems

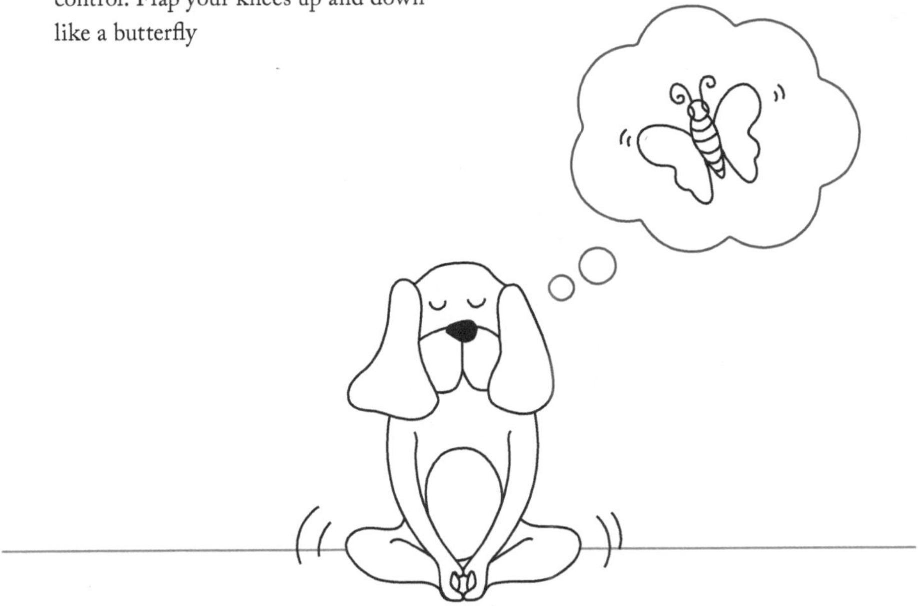

05 – TWO MINUTES

dancer

instructions

1 Stand up. Bending the right leg at the knee, grab your big toe and pull it towards the head

2 Stay in this position for a few seconds, fixing your gaze at a point in front of you to maintain balance. Focus on controlled breathing to steady the posture

3 Repeat on the other side

benefits

1 Builds balance

2 Builds focus and concentration (so kids can crack those exams)

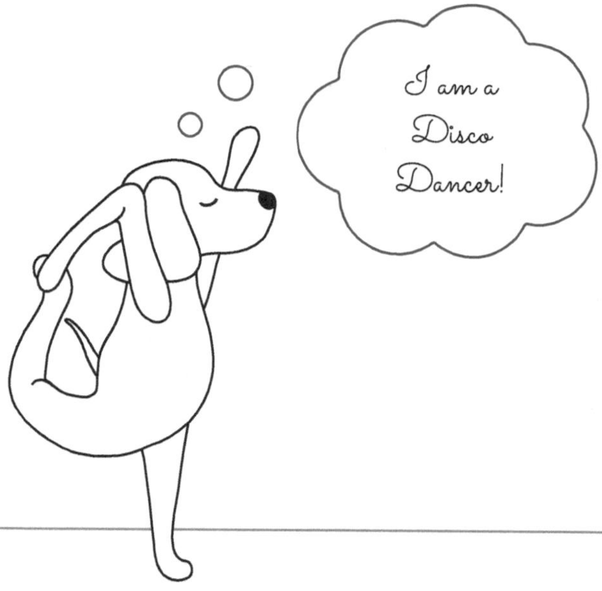

yoga nidra

Yoga nidra is an excellent technique for kids to ease pre-exam or pre-competition tension, which is getting worse and worse these days. It's a great way to relax physically, mentally and emotionally.

instructions

1 Lie down in Shavasana. Spend a few minutes paying attention to your breath and relaxing your body and mind

2 You now have to focus on each part of your body, starting from your toes and moving up to your head

3 Focus on your toes. Bring your attention to your toes. Scrunch them up. Release

4 Now tense up both your feet. Life them an inch off the ground. Bring them down. Relax

5 Focus on the muscles in your calves. Tense them up. Relax

6 Focus on your knees. Bring your attention to your knees. Relax

7 Focus on both your legs. Tense them up. Lift them an inch off the ground. Relax

8 Focus on your tummy. Tense up all your tummy muscles. Relax

9 Focus on your back. Feel your back muscles. Relax

10 Scrunch your shoulders up to your ears. Tense them up. Relax

11 Make your hands into tight fists. Squeeze all the muscles in your arms. Raise your arms an inch off the ground. Relax

12 Close your eyes. Scrunch your nose, forehead and lips, making a small ball of your face. Open your mouth, make a sighing sound. Relax

13 Take a few seconds to pay attention to every part of your body and relax. Stay in Savasana for a few minutes. Relax

benefits

1 Great for hips and knees (prevents serious injuries from all those falls)

It's good to keep mixing things up for kids. Check out *My Book of Yoga*, my book for kids, for more yoga asanas.

yoga for travellers

Travelling is strenuous both on your body and your mind. Being stuck in a seat for hours, in unnatural conditions – regulated cabin pressures and breathing in stale air – can take a huge toll on your systems. This is why you are often cranky and tired after long flights, even though you have just been sitting. If you are travelling internationally, jet lag particularly can be a menace. Luckily, yoga can help limit the impact of travelling on short or long-haul flights. This 10-minute routine can help you fight fatigue, relax tight and constricted muscles, regain balance, oxygenate a starved body and get your sleep cycle back on track. You can even do some parts of this routine in transit whilst flying.

your notes:

01 – TWO MINUTES

kapalabhati

REFER TO PAGE 154

This is the perfect kriya to do because it stimulates your respiratory systems and the retention of breath is also crucial because it helps with oxygenation.

your notes:

02 – TWO MINUTES

anulom vilom

PRANAYAMA

REFER TO PAGE 76

your notes:

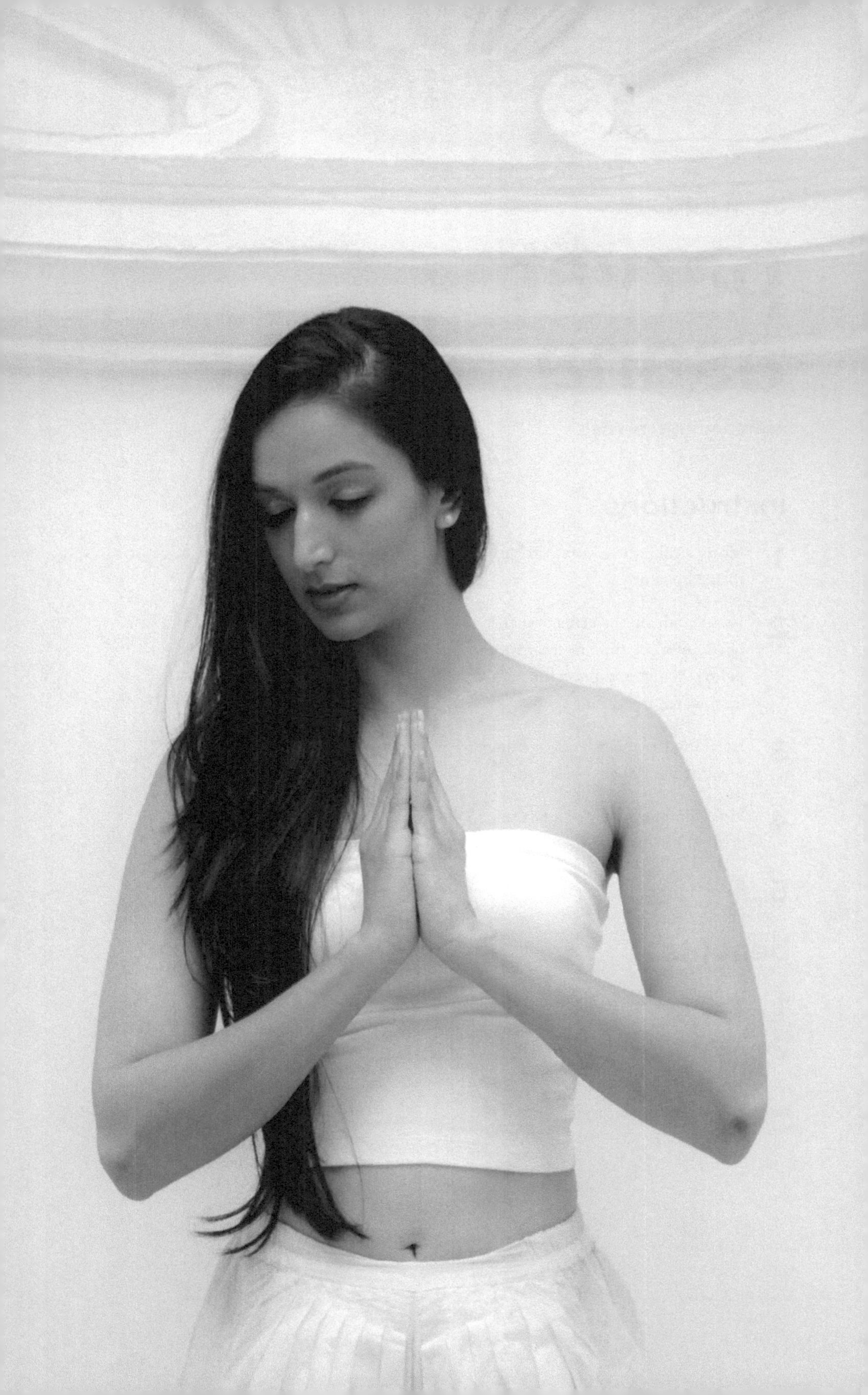

03 – TWO MINUTES

parvat asana

SEATED MOUNTAIN POSE

instructions

1. Sit up straight in a comfortable, relaxed posture
2. Inhale, raising the arms over the head, interlace the fingers, turn the palms around and press the palms up towards the ceiling
3. Relaxing the shoulders, gaze upward towards the fingers
4. Hold for a few counts and exhale to bring the arms back down
5. Repeat

benefits

1. Relieves tension in the back
2. Stretches the spine

contraindications: Neck injury

YOGA TIP:
You can do this asana anytime, anywhere, even on the plane! Just make sure your spine is straight.

Relax,
Yoga,
Breathe.

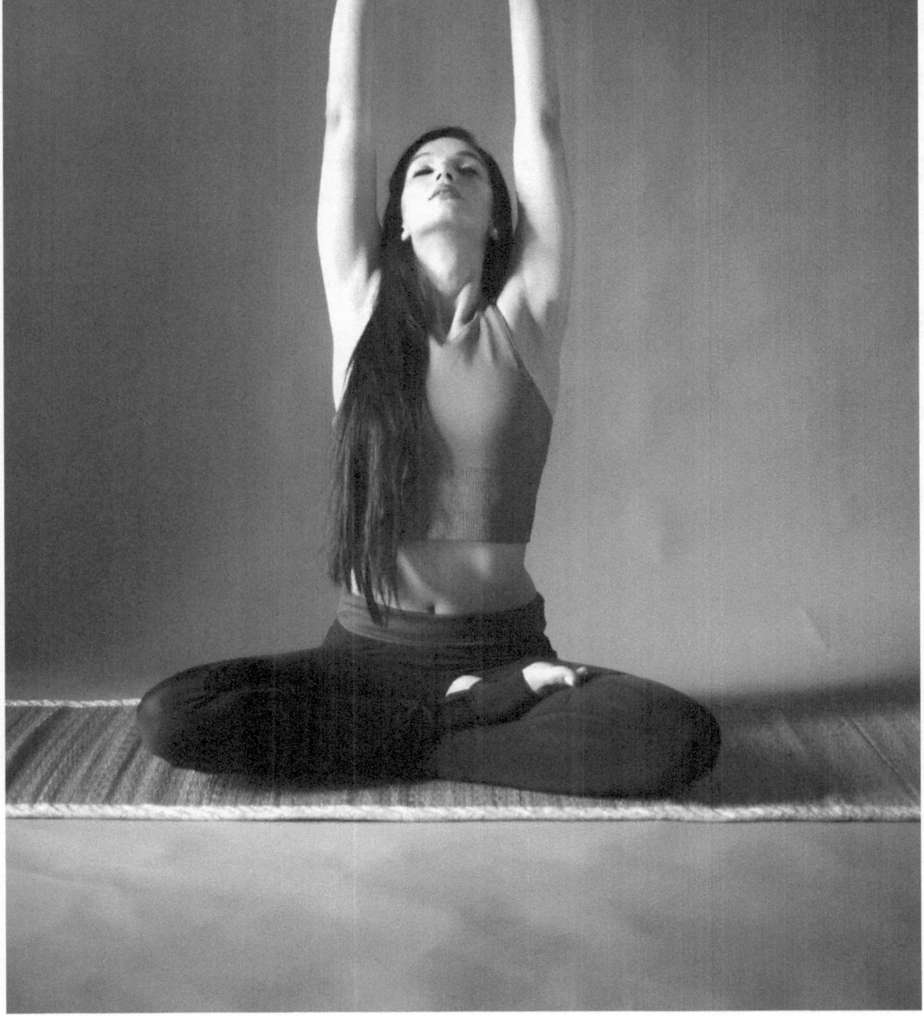

04 – TWO MINUTES

kapotasana

PIGEON POSE

instructions

1. Begin by coming up on your arms and legs
2. Stretch the left leg out and point the toes towards the back. Slide the right foot towards the left hand so the knee is pointing to the front.
3. Stay here and breathe, sinking deeper and stretching the pelvis and legs
4. Inhale and bring the chin to the ground
5. Exhale, lift the chin and repeat on the other side

benefits

1. Relieves tension from extended periods of sitting
2. Relieves tension in the hips, stretches the chest and back

contraindications: Knee injuries, hip injuries

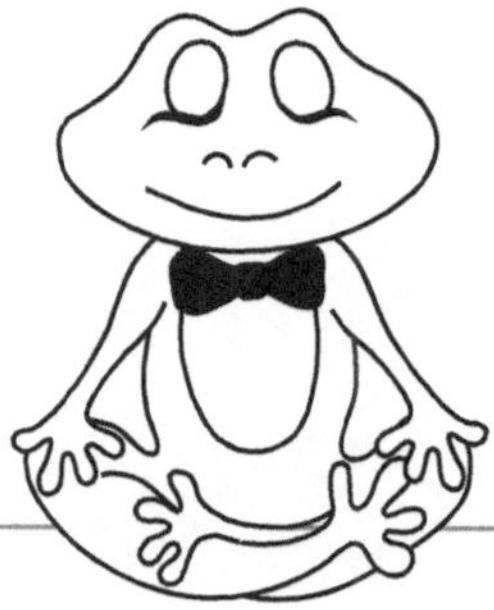

your notes:

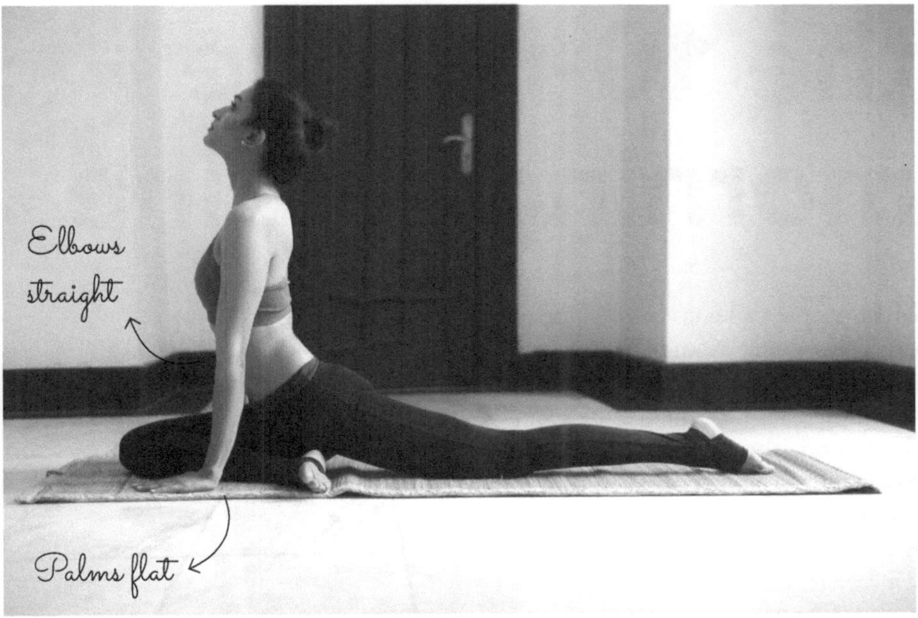

05 – ONE MINUTE

sasangasana

RABBIT POSE

REFER TO PAGE 34

your notes:

---

06 – ONE MINUTE

shavasana

IT'S VERY IMPORTANT FOR TRAVELLERS TO DO SHAVASANA TO RELAX THE SPINE!

REFER TO PAGE 28

the 10-minute morning routine

Most people wake up in the morning, run a few quick errands, chug a cup of tea, gobble some toast and rush to work. There is no time to think, no time to breathe and certainly no time to do yoga. The fact remains that even a short 10-minute routine can vastly improve your day. It can kick-start your metabolism, stretch out your muscles, oxygenate your body, get your hormones functioning in the proper way and make you feel 200 per cent better overall. The best part is that the positive effect of yoga lasts not just in that moment, but for the rest of the day.

Here is a simple, effective and complete solution to get your morning started off right.

your notes:

01 – FIVE MINUTES

surya namaskar

REFER TO PAGE 96

I start my day off with the namaskar. Even if I don't get time to do my full yoga routine, I make sure to do at least 3 rounds of Surya Namaskar to open up my body. They are a complete workout and work on all parts of your body. If you coordinate each step with your breath, you get the benefits of a pranayama practise as well.

You should be able to complete 3 rounds in 5 minutes. If you want a more vigorous workout, do 6 rounds of this, 6 on each leg.

02 – TWO MINUTES

kapalabhati

REFER TO PAGE 16

YOGA TIP:
Before starting this routine, drink a cup of hot water with some lemon, honey and ginger. It helps create an alkaline environment in your body thereby reducing its acidity. It is detoxifying and energizing and helps makes you less susceptible to disease and illness.

This is my secret and I start my morning like this every day.

There is a lot of confusion about how to do a Surya Namaskar correctly and lots of people are afraid for they think the routine might injure their knees or their back. If you do the practise correctly, you don't have to worry at all.

03 – TWO MINUTES

anulom vilom

PRANAYAMA

REFER TO PAGE 76

your notes:

04 – ONE MINUTE

shavasana

CORPSE POSE

REFER TO PAGE 28

your notes:

night-time routine

It can be deeply beneficial to do a quick 10-minute routine before you head to bed, especially if you have trouble sleeping. This short practise will help ease your body and mind into a deeper and more restful sleep. Yoga accentuates the quality of your sleep over the quantity of hours you think you may be resting. Just 10-minutes of yoga can help reduce your sleeping time by up to 2 hours.

your notes:

01 – TWO MINUTES

vajrasana

WITH DEEP BREATHING

instructions

1 Begin in Vajrasana

2 Breathe in deeply, for a count of 1, 2, 3, 4, 5, 6, 7, 8. Breathe out completely for a count of 1, 2, 3, 4, 5, 6, 7, 8. As you breathe, focus on the energy point between your forehead

benefits

1 Deeply relaxing and rejuvenating

contraindications: Knee injuries

YOGA FACT:
Vajrasana is fantastic for digestion. Make sure you sit in Vajrasana after dinner. If you experience any discomfort in your knees, you may use a cushion to elevate your pelvis and relieve any strain on the knees.

These mountains that you are carrying, you were only supposed to climb.

- Najwa Zebian

02 – TWO MINUTES

gomukh asana

COW FACE POSE

REFER TO PAGE 72

benefits

1 Relaxes the hips and shoulders

2 Calms the mind

contraindications: Knee injuries, neck injuries, shoulder pain.

your notes:

03 – TWO MINUTES

balasana

CHILD'S POSE

REFER TO PAGE 118

04 – TWO MINUTES

supta matsyendra asana

SUPINE TWIST

instructions

1. Lie on the back with the arms on either side of the body
2. Bending the right knee at a 90-degree angle, place it on the floor next to the left knee
3. Extending the arms out to the side, gaze towards the right hand
4. Exhale and repeat on the other side

benefits

1. Increases circulation
2. Relieves tension in the lower back
3. Relieves tension in the intercostal muscles (muscles between the ribs)

contraindications: None!

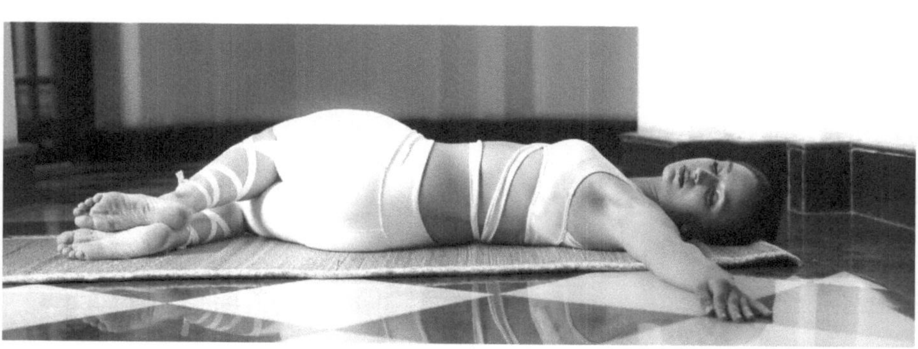

05 – TWO MINUTES

yoga nidra

REFER TO PAGE 177

Yoga nidra, fondly known as yogic sleep, is a powerful tool for activating the subconscious. In addition to being the perfect relaxation tool to winding down after a busy day, yoga nidra can be used to help your mind further your goals and aspirations. Before you begin yoga nidra, you can focus briefly on or think of a task you would like to achieve.

Yoga is the journey of the self, through the self, to the self.

your notes:

yoga for sinus infections and colds

When you have a sinus infection or a cold, the last thing that you want to do is to get out of bed, but simple yoga asanas help bring your body back to health and will help you feel better faster. Simple inversions and stretches stimulate your lymphatic system, which cleanses your body, ridding it of lingering viruses. While yoga asanas that use gentle twists increase the blood flow to the spleen which help fight infection and cleanse the blood.

your notes:

01 – TWO MINUTES

kapalabhati

Practice up to 3 rounds for a total of 2 minutes

REFER TO PAGE 16

your notes:

02 – TWO MINUTES

surya bheda

PRANAYAMA

REFER TO PAGE 130

your notes:

The heat-generating aspect of Surya Bheda pranayama is great for getting rid of colds.

YOGA FACT:

Sinus problems are usually worsened by stress, which releases hormones and histamines that trigger inflammation. Relaxation diminishes the fight or flight response and reduces allergic symptoms.

03 – TWO MINUTES

seated chest lift

instructions

1 Sit up straight in a comfortable, relaxed posture

2 Move the arms behind the body and press the fingertips into the ground

3 Inhale and lift the chest up

4 Stay here and breath focussing on the breath

5 To deepen the stretch, lift the hips creating even more length in the spine

6 Exhale and slowly lower the hips to the ground

benefits

1 Alleviates tension in the neck, shoulders, back and spine

2 Stretches the chest muscles

contraindications: None!

04 – TWO MINUTES

padahastasana

WITH ELBOW HOLD

REFER TO PAGE 82

06 – TWO MINUTES

viparita karani

LEGS UP IN THE AIR

instructions

1 Sit up straight in a comfortable, relaxed posture, facing the wall

2 Shifting the pelvis as close to the wall as possible, place the legs up against the wall

3 Inhale and exhale, relaxing deeper into the posture

benefits

1 Relieves tension on the spine and back

contraindications: Vertigo

YOGA TIP:
For an additional challenge you can avoid the wall and just bring your legs up.

Place a bolster or towel under your head or hips to make it a little bit more comfortable.

your notes:

05 – TWO MINUTES

balasana

CHILD'S POSE

REFER TO PAGE 118

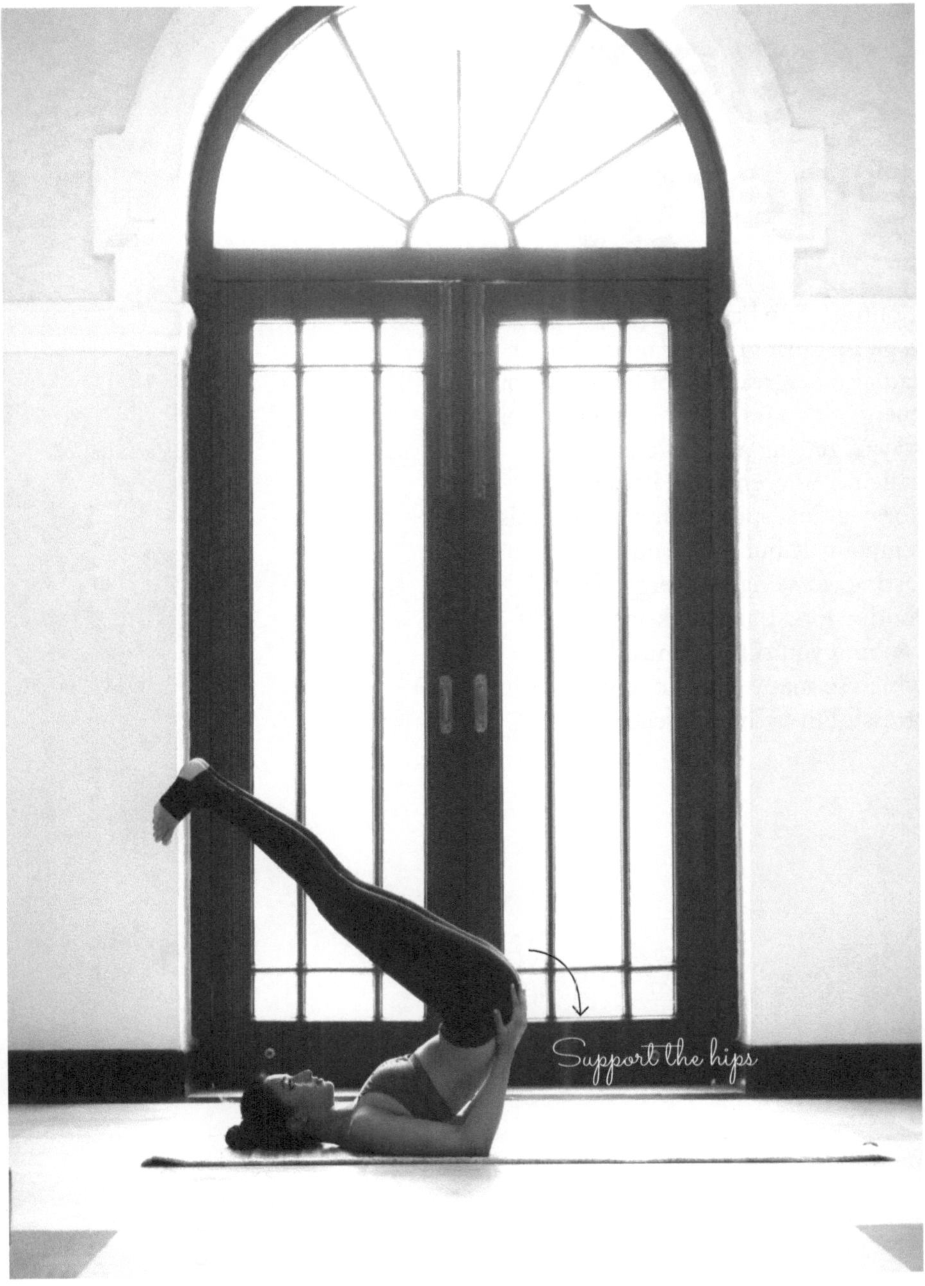
Support the hips

yoga for energy

Contrary to what some people think, yoga isn't just great for relaxation, it can also be great way of boosting your energy. It's a far better (and healthier) way of getting a jolt of energy than caffeine, or even a jog, because it does not just spike your energy levels temporarily but gives you long-lasting, sustainable energy. Try this routine for a quick pick-me-up or if you find yourself chronically tired, which so many of us do, given the stressful lives that we lead.

your notes:

01 – THREE MINUTES

kapalabhati

REFER TO PAGE 16

benefits

1. Improves blood circulation
2. Increases oxygenation
3. Strengthens the lungs

contraindications: Major respiratory disorders

your notes:

Open up and say Om.

02 – TWO MINUTES

anulom vilom

PRANAYAMA

REFER TO PAGE 76

your notes:

03 – TWO MINUTES

druta halasana

DYNAMIC PLOUGH POSE

instructions

1. Lie flat on the back with arms on either side of the body
2. With controlled momentum, swing the legs over the head
3. Placing the palms firmly on the ground, inhale and exhale deeply reaching for the ground with the legs as far as is possible
4. Roll back to a seated posture with the legs extended straight out in front of you
5. Inhale and exhale, moving into a forward bend bringing the forehead towards the knees
6. Return to a seated posture. This is one round
7. Continue for 2 minutes
8. To counterbalance this pose, sit in Vajrasana for 10 seconds

benefits

1. Regulates the thyroid gland
2. Relieves stress and fatigue
3. Increases metabolism

contraindications: Spinal injuries, back injuries, neck injuries, high blood pressure, pregnancy

your notes:

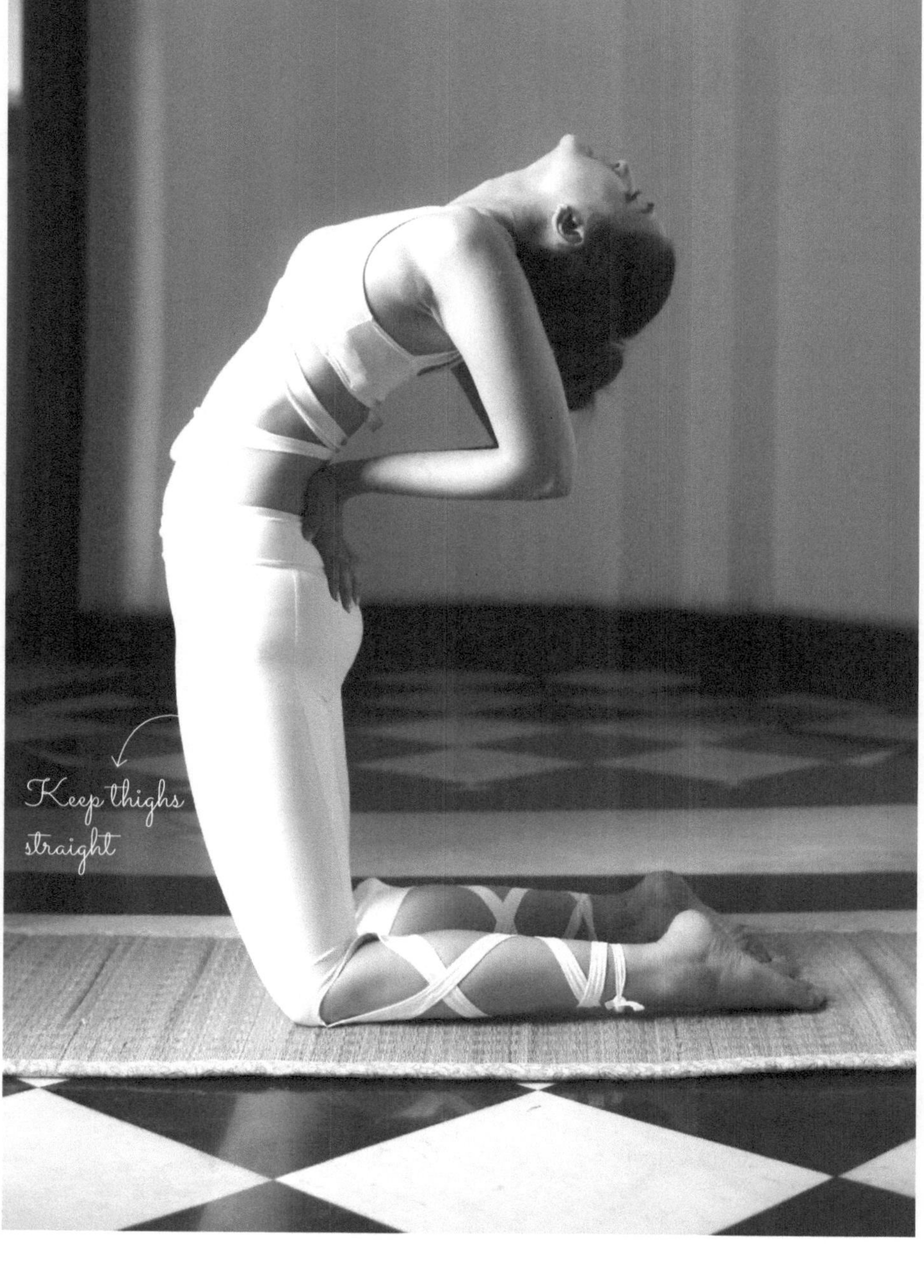
Keep thighs straight

04 – ONE MINUTE

ustrasana

CAMEL POSE

instructions

1. Start in a kneeling position with the hands on the lower back for support
2. Slowly bend backwards, engaging the core
3. Drop the head back and tilt the chin towards the ceiling, continuing to breath

benefits

1. Stimulates digestion
2. Strengthens the entire spine
3. Relieves pain in the lower back

contraindications: Neck injuries, spinal injuries

The very heart of yoga practise is abhyasa – steady effort in the direction you want to go.

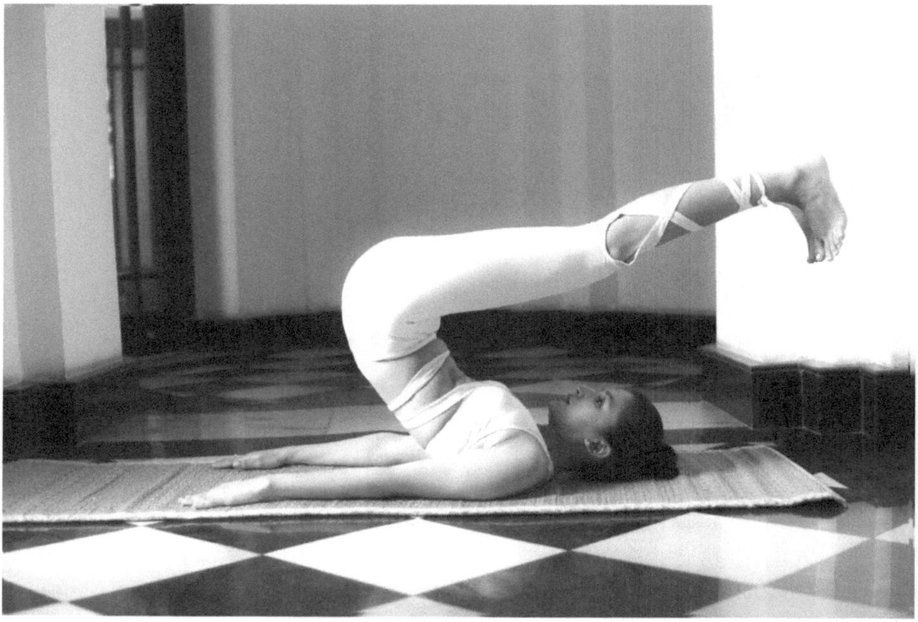

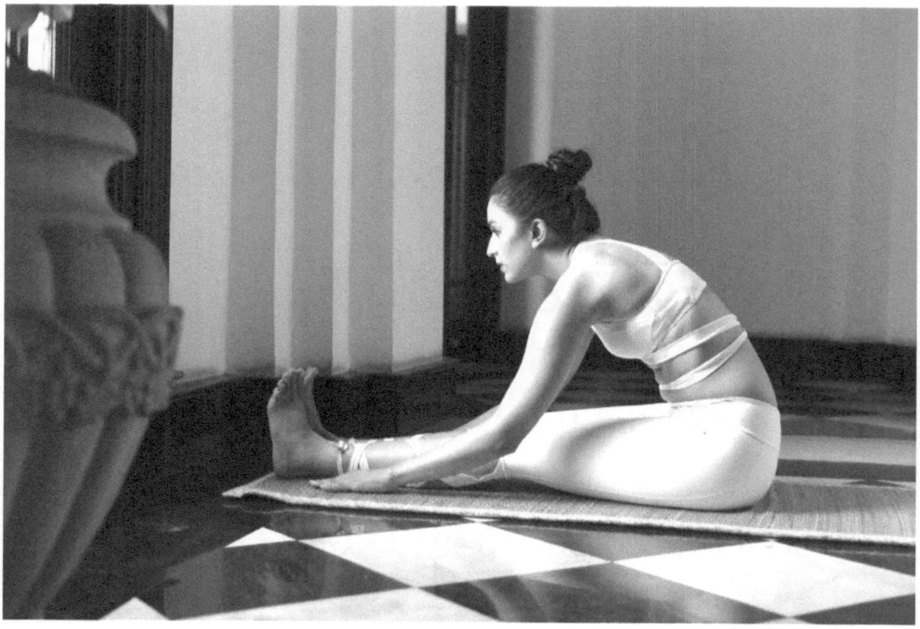

05 – ONE MINUTE

dhanurasana

BOW POSE

REFER TO PAGE 48

YOGA FACT:
The Dhanurasana gives a beautiful stretch to the spine as well as a massage to your digestive organs. It wakes up the body.

your notes:

05 – ONE MINUTE

shavasana

CORPSE POSE

REFER TO PAGE 28

your notes:

yoga for fasting

Fasting is meant to go hand in hand with the spiritual practises of prayer and meditation. As you detach from food and the sense of taste, you focus inwards. Religious fasting is also great for your health. Both the Navratras fall during the change of season when it is advised that one should eat less and detoxify as this prevents disease and illness, something you are more susceptible to during this specific time of the year.

There are all sorts of fasts. Some people only do fruits, other people do phalari, which means they take out grains from their diet while others do only juice or water. I, for example, try to fast one day a week. On this day, I only eat fruits and boiled vegetables without any salt. It's a great way to give your body a break and while it can be hard, the next day I am always glad I did it. Any sort of fast can make you feel low on energy, weak, tired and cranky. Yoga is a wonderful way to beat these symptoms. Even simple asanas can help drive away fatigue, and help you feel more relaxed and calm.

your notes:

01 – FIVE MINUTES

meditation basics

BASIC BEGINNER'S MEDITATION

There are all sorts of meditations out there and so many different books say so many different things. Some say meditate with your eyes open, others say to meditate with them closed. Some endorse meditation while walking, others say sleep is the best form of mediation. There are so many theories and practises that it can often get confusing, and then you don't want to meditate at all. Worry no more, here is a basic beginners' meditation that is easy to follow.

instructions

1. Sit up straight in a comfortable, relaxed posture
2. Resting both hands on the knees, bring together the thumb and forefinger in Gyan mudra
3. Inhale deeply and exhale completely, extending your breath as you go along
4. As you breathe, try to focus on your breath and clear your mind of all wavering thoughts
5. Focus on silencing your mind by remaining focused on your breath. If thoughts are flooding the mind, observe them and allow them to pass by without passing judgement or developing any attachment to them
6. Stay here for 5 minutes, bringing your mind to your breath every time it wavers
7. Voila! It's as simple as that

benefits

1. Calms the body and mind
2. Increases oxygenation
3. Sharpens mental focus

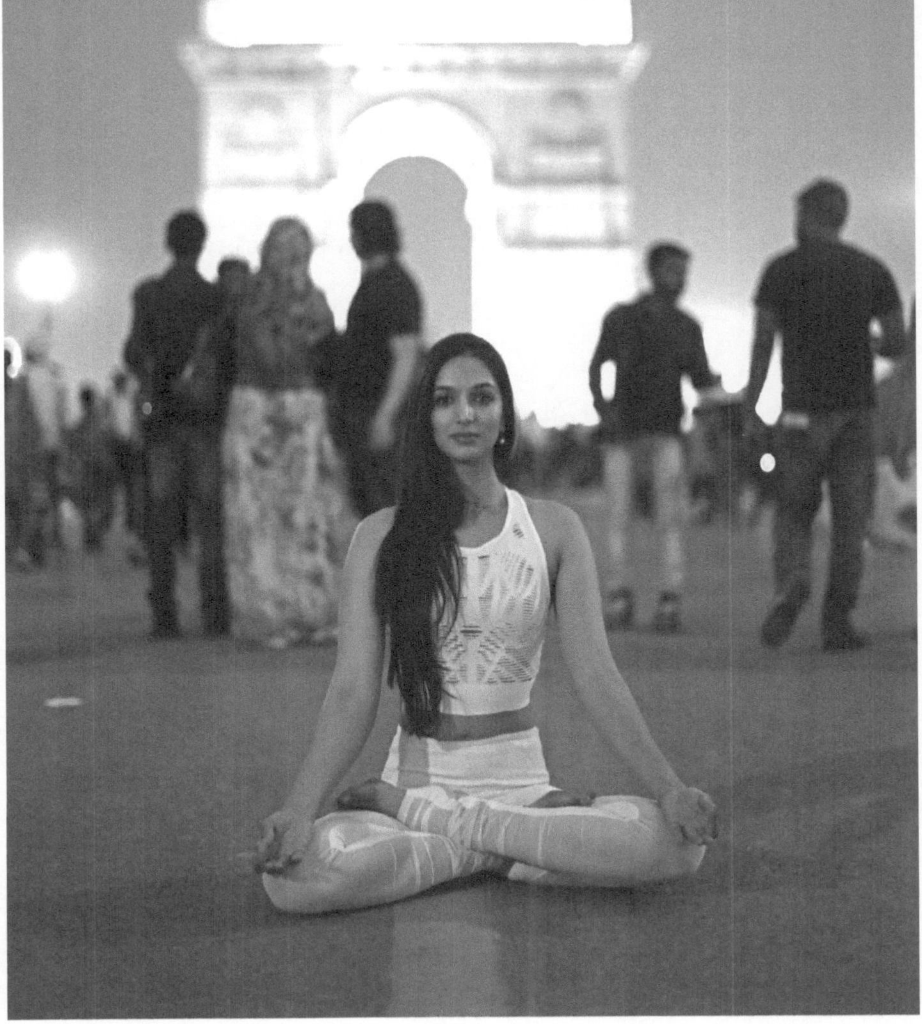

02 – TWO MINUTES

sheetali pranayama

REFER TO PAGE 94

YOGA TIP:

Meditation is best practised as soon as you wake up. The second-best option is to practise it just before you go to bed. The absolute best option is to practise it both as soon as you wake up and then before you go to bed for 5 minutes each.

In the beginning, even 5 minutes will feel like torture but slowly, over time, things will become much easier and even enjoyable.

your notes:

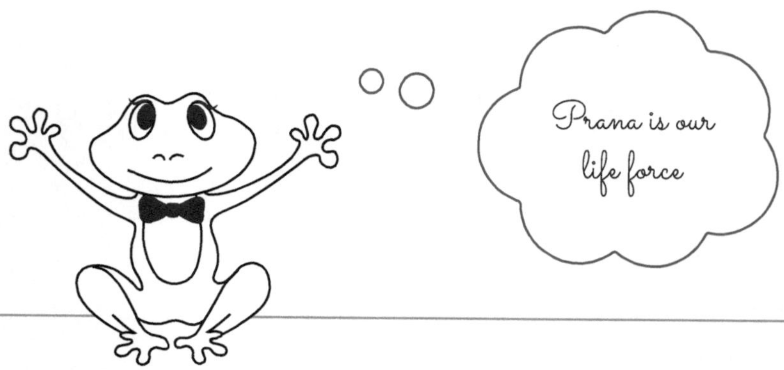

03 – ONE MINUTE

parivrtta sukhasana

SEATED SPINAL TWIST

REFER TO PAGE 18

*Yoga is like life.
It is the balance of holding
on and letting go.*

your notes:

04 – ONE MINUTE

hindolasana

BABY CRADLE POSE

instructions

1 Sit up straight in a comfortable, relaxed posture with the legs stretched out in front

2 Lift the right leg placing the right sole against the inside of the left elbow, and the right knee inside the right elbow begin to sway from left to right gently. Don't forget to breathe

3 Release the right leg. Repeat on the other side

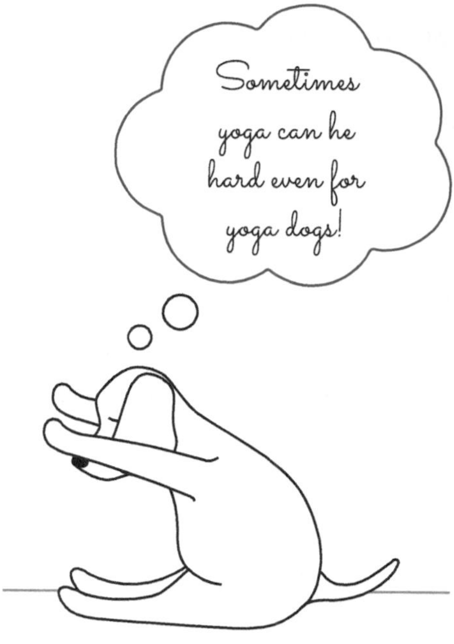

benefits

1 Stimulates digestion during fasting

2 Stretch for the legs and hips

contraindications: Knee injuries

your notes:

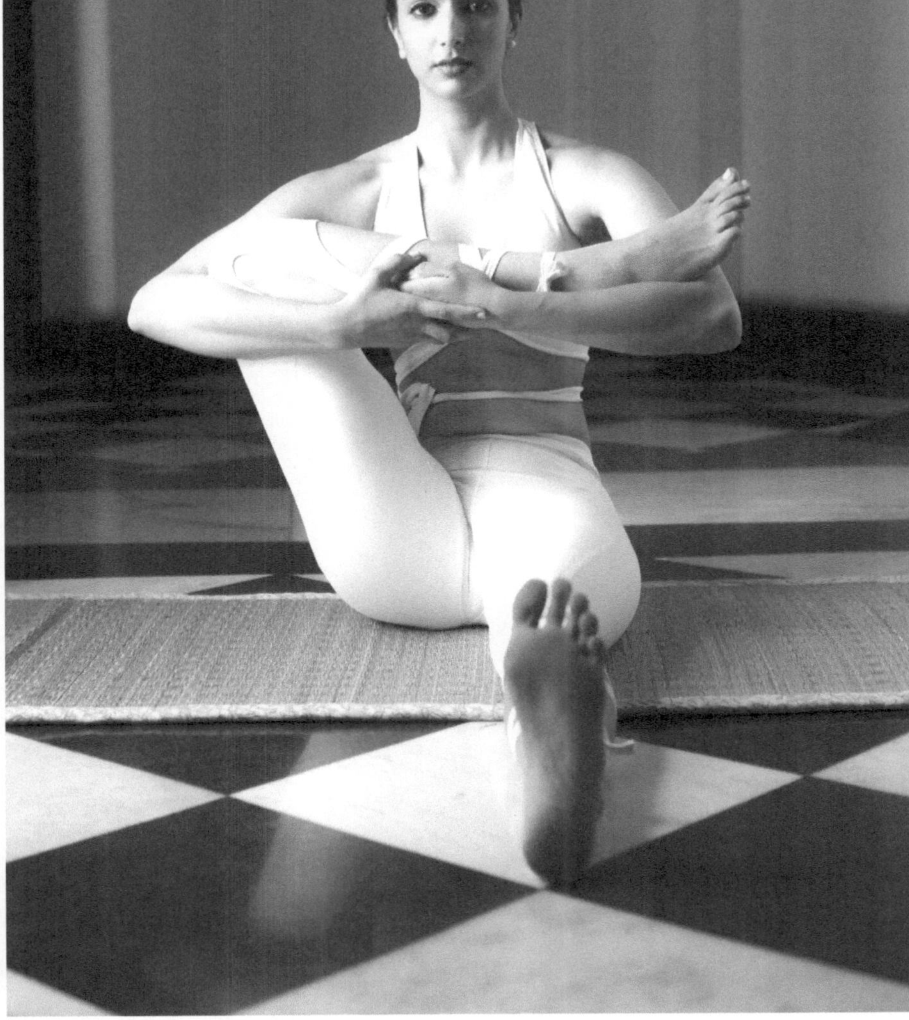

05 – ONE MINUTE

pawan mukta asana

THE ROCK

instructions

1. Lying down on your back, bring both knees to the chest
2. Place the palms on the knees and gently rock from side to side massaging the sides of the body
3. Continue rocking gently and focus on steadying the breath

benefits

1. Gives a gentle massage to the back and spine
2. Helps in circulation
3. Relaxes the whole body
4. Feels good!

contraindications: None

your notes:

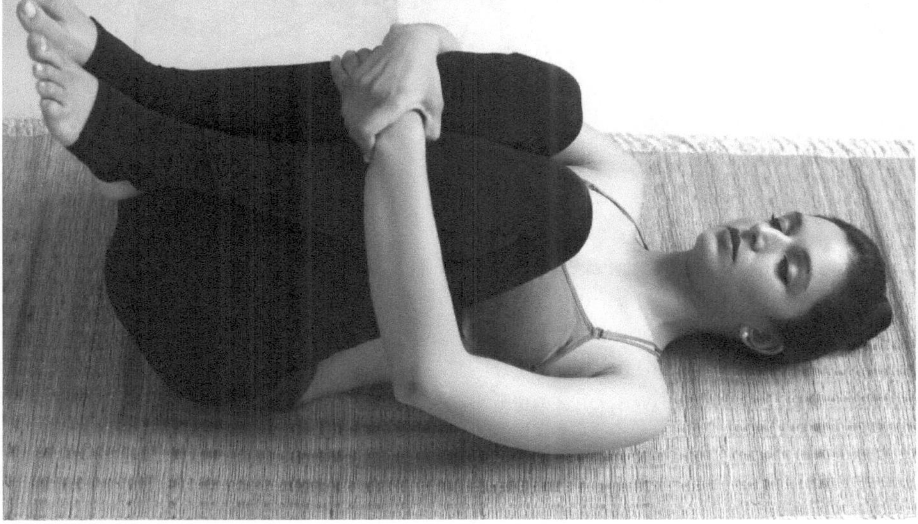

Yoga is like music.
The rhythm of the body,
the melody of the mind
and the harmony of the soul,
create the symphony of life.

– BKS Iyengar

yoga for binge eating

Even the best amongst you have, at some point in your lives, indulged in binge eating. It often happens on days when work is taxing, during stressful times in our personal lives, or sometimes when you are too relaxed, like on holiday. One sure-shot effect of binge eating is how gross you feel afterwards. And you desperately wish to rewind the clock and make healthier choices. Well, now you can. Doing just 10-minutes of yoga will not only help you feel a *lot* better after binge eating, but will also help you control it, especially if this is something of a regular habit.

your notes:

01 – TWO MINUTES

sheetkari pranayama

REFER TO PAGE 92

02 – TWO MINUTES

urdhva mukha svanasana

DOWNWARD DOG

REFER TO PAGE 106

03 – TWO MINUTES

anjaneya asana

WARRIOR POSE ONE

REFER TO PAGE 108

04 – TWO MINUTES

trikonasana

TRIANGLE POSE

REFER TO PAGE 150

05 – ONE MINUTE

balasana

CHILD'S POSE

REFER TO PAGE 118

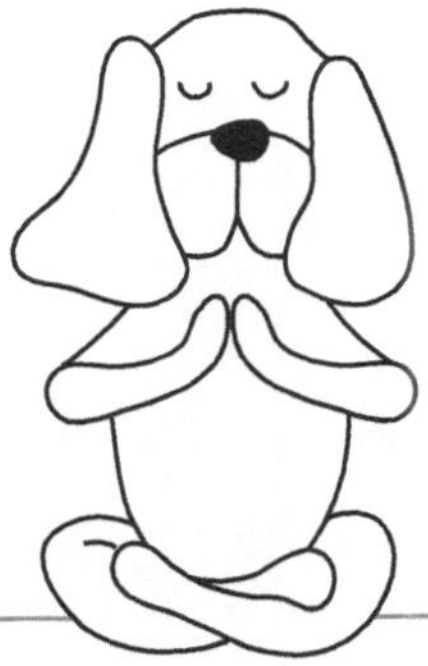

your notes:

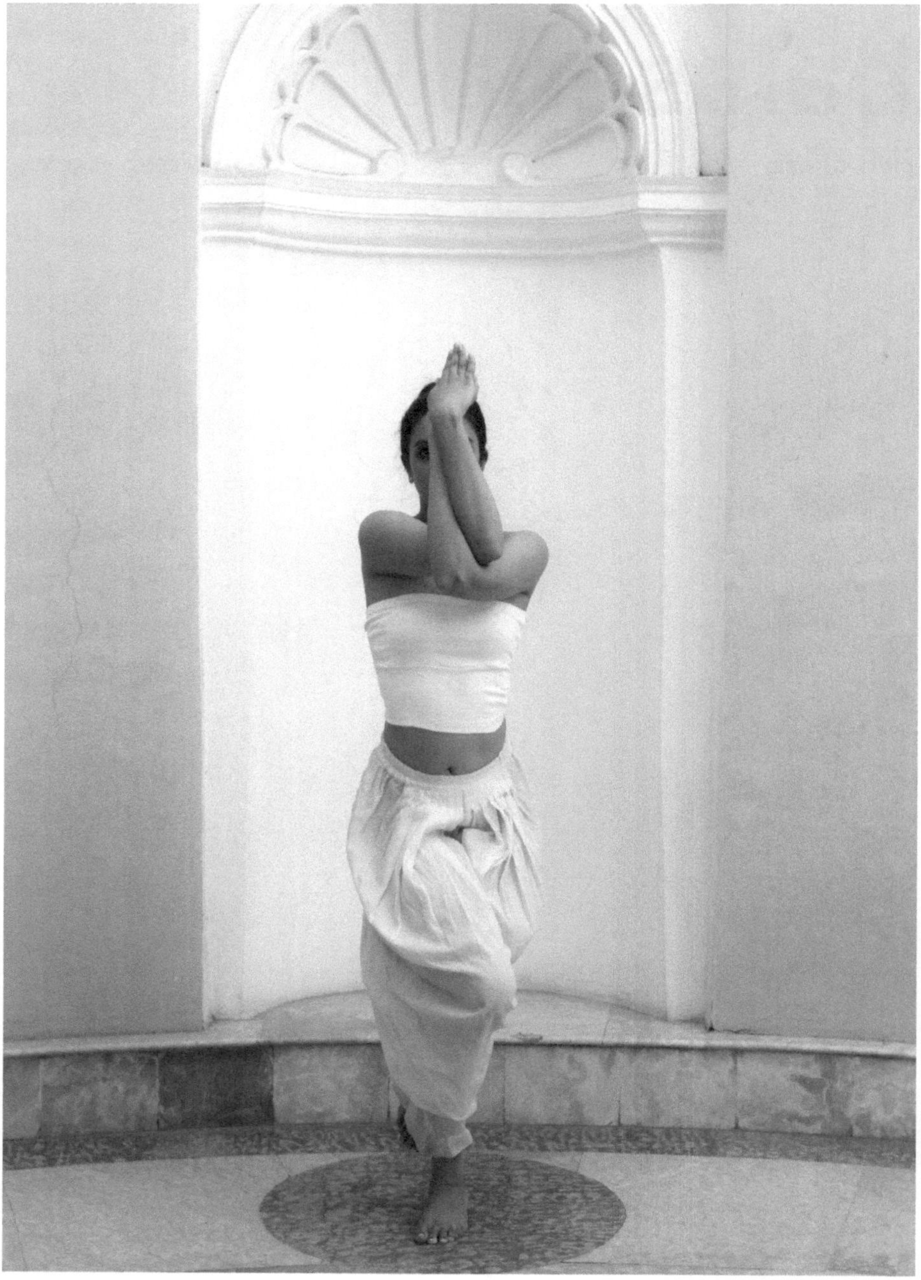

06 – ONE MINUTE

garuda asana

THE EAGLE

instructions

1 Stand up straight with the feet hip distance apart and the arms on either side of the body

2 Bending slightly at the knees, place the right leg over the left knee, hooking the right foot on the calf or ankle

3 Wrap the arms around each other and bring the palms in prayer position. Wrap the right arm over the left arm

4 Inhale and ground your feet into the floor. As you exhale sink deeper into the pose, bending more at the knees

5 Exhale and return to a standing position

6 Repeat on the other side placing the left leg over the right knee. Switch arms

benefits

1 Builds mental focus

2 Relieves pain in the lower back

contraindications: Knee injuries

YOGA TIP:
Fix your gaze upon a point as this will help you maintain balance. This asana can be very easy if you relax into the asana.

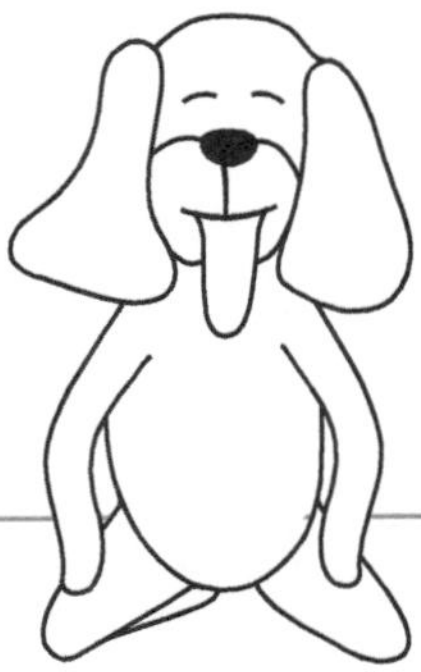

yoga for eyes

In this electronic age of computers, smart phones and television, your eyes are more strained than ever before. You may not feel the need to exercise your eyes today, but if you want to protect yourself from blurry vision in the future, these simple eye-yoga exercises are a fantastic way of maintaining long-term health for all age groups. Your eyes are made up of muscles, and just like other muscles, you can work with these to keep problems away.

your notes:

01 – TWO MINUTES

bhramari pranayama

HUMMING BEE BREATH

instructions

1. Sit up straight in a comfortable, relaxed posture
2. Sealing the ears with the index fingers raise the elbows slightly out on either side
3. Inhale and exhale hum loudly as if emulating a bee

benefits

1. Relaxes the eyes
2. Alleviates symptoms of migraines
3. Improves concentration and memory

contraindications: None

YOGA FACT:
In her book *Eye Yoga: How You See is How You Think*, Jane Rigney Battenberg says eye muscles are eight times stronger than they need to be and thus they don't need to be strengthened as much as stretched, relaxed and fine-tuned. You will need to balance between the stretching and strengthening exercises, where the eyes learn to work and see together while being able to relax and loosen to re-pattern the coordination between the brain and the eyes.

your notes:

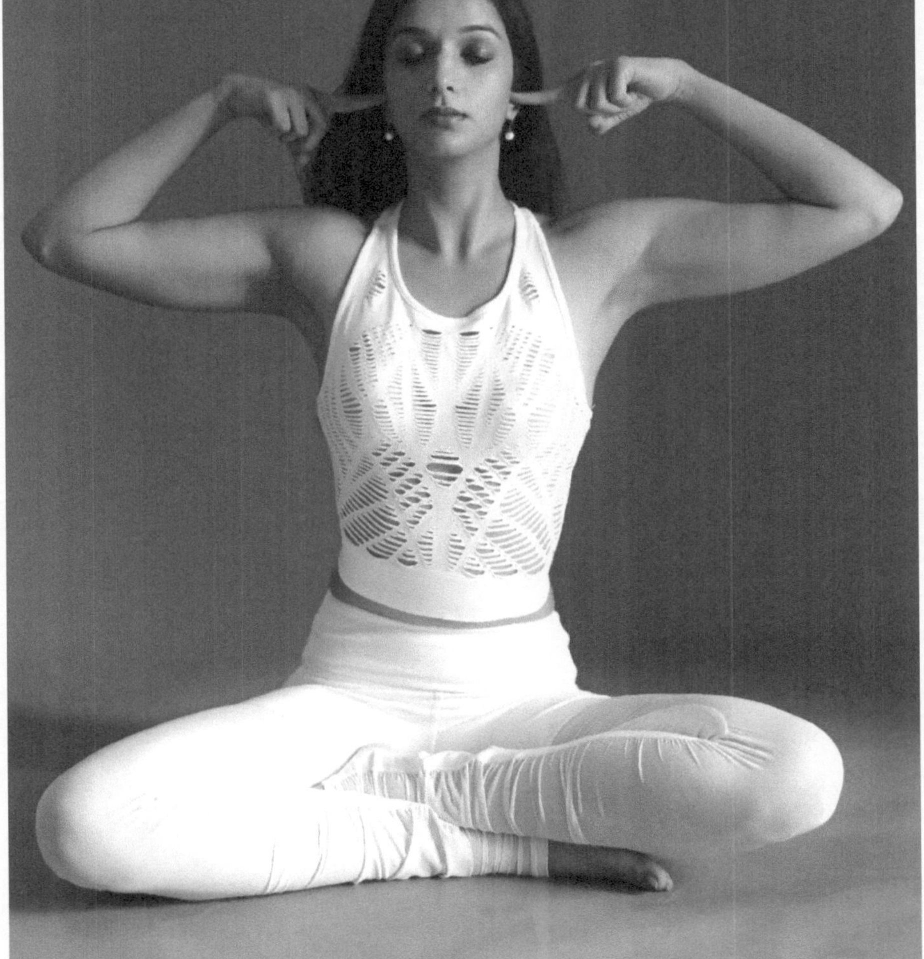

02 – TWO MINUTES

blinking and cupping

instructions

1 Rub the palms together until you feel them warm up

2 Cup the eyes by placing the base of the palms over the eyes for ten seconds

3 Remove the palms

4 Blink as you look up, down, left, right and forward. Blink 10 times in each direction. This is one round

5 Repeat twice

YOGA TIP:
The *easiest* way of keeping the eyes healthy is to blink! So, blink away, as often as you can.

benefits

1 Cleans debris from the eyes and prevents infection

2 Stimulates circulation to the eye area and surrounding nerves

3 Protects eye tissue

contraindications: Remove glasses and contact lenses before practising this exercise

your notes:

03 – TWO MINUTES

eye movements

instructions

1. Sit up straight in a comfortable, relaxed posture
2. Keeping the spine straight, look up towards the ceiling and blink. Look to the nose, blink Look to the left, blink. Look to the right, blink. This is one round
3. Roll the eyes clockwise, blink. Roll the eyes anti-clockwise, blink
4. Cup the eyes gently with the hands

your notes:

04 – TWO MINUTES

eye movements

WITH HAND MOVEMENTS

instructions

1. Sit up straight in a comfortable, relaxed posture
2. Extend both the arms out straight in front with hands in a thumbs-up position
3. Direct the gaze toward the thumb as you move the arm to the right till it is in line with the shoulder
4. Bring the arm back to centre
5. Repeat with the left arm

benefits

1. Strengthens and stretches the muscles of the eyes
2. Cures myopia (short-sightedness)
3. Cures hypermetropia (far-sightedness)

contraindications: Recent eye surgery, glaucoma

Tend to your inner sanctuary.

05 – ONE MINUTE

bhujangasana

COBRA POSE

REFER TO PAGE 80

If you want a more involved movement to round up your exercise, then you can replace one of the above exercises with Bhujangasana. When you draw your chin up towards the ceiling, move your eyes up and fix your gaze at a point. You can even look at the tip of your nose. Try not to blink.

your notes:

06 – ONE MINUTE

balasana

CHILD'S POSE

REFER TO PAGE 118

This asana brings blood to the eyes leading to better circulation and relaxation.

07 – TWO MINUTES

trataka

YOGIC GAZING

instructions

1. Sit up straight in a comfortable, relaxed posture
2. Place an object, preferably a candle, 2 feet away
3. Continue breathing and focus the gaze on the object without blinking for as long as possible until the eyes begin to water

benefits

1. Improves vision, focus and memory
2. Strengthens concentration
3. Develops willpower

contraindications: Eye surgeries, eye injuries

YOGA TIP:
Keep the room dimly lit. You will be able to concentrate better, almost as if in meditation.

your notes:

yoga for focus and concentration

Is your mind all over the place all the time? When you're supposed to be writing an email, are you instead checking your Facebook or WhatsApp? A hectic lifestyle without any time for observing can lead to an unfocused mind and poor concentration. Yoga can help fix this. With these simple asanas, done for a short 10 minutes every day, you will not just stabilize a wobbly mind but also sharpen and strengthen it. The act of physically balancing yourself can, and will, lead to mental balance. Also, when you focus your mind during your asana practise you will find it easier to focus during the day.

your notes:

01 – TWO MINUTES

anulom vilom

PRANAYAMA

REFER TO PAGE 76

YOGA TIP:
Most of us never live in the present moment, instead we are always thinking about either the past or the future. Being in the present moment is not just good for overall mental and emotional health but can also lead to greater productivity. Asanas work by bringing you back to the present moment and help practice mindfulness.

02 – TWO MINUTES

vrikshasana

TREE POSE

instructions

1 Stand up straight with the feet hip distance apart and the arms on either side of the body

2 Place the left foot on the inner right thigh, inhale and raise the arms above the head joining the palms

3 Balance on the left foot and direct the gaze at a fixed point

4 Repeat on the other side

benefits

1 Improves focus and concentration

2 Strengthens the leg muscles

3 Improves alignment

contraindications: Knee injuries, back injuries

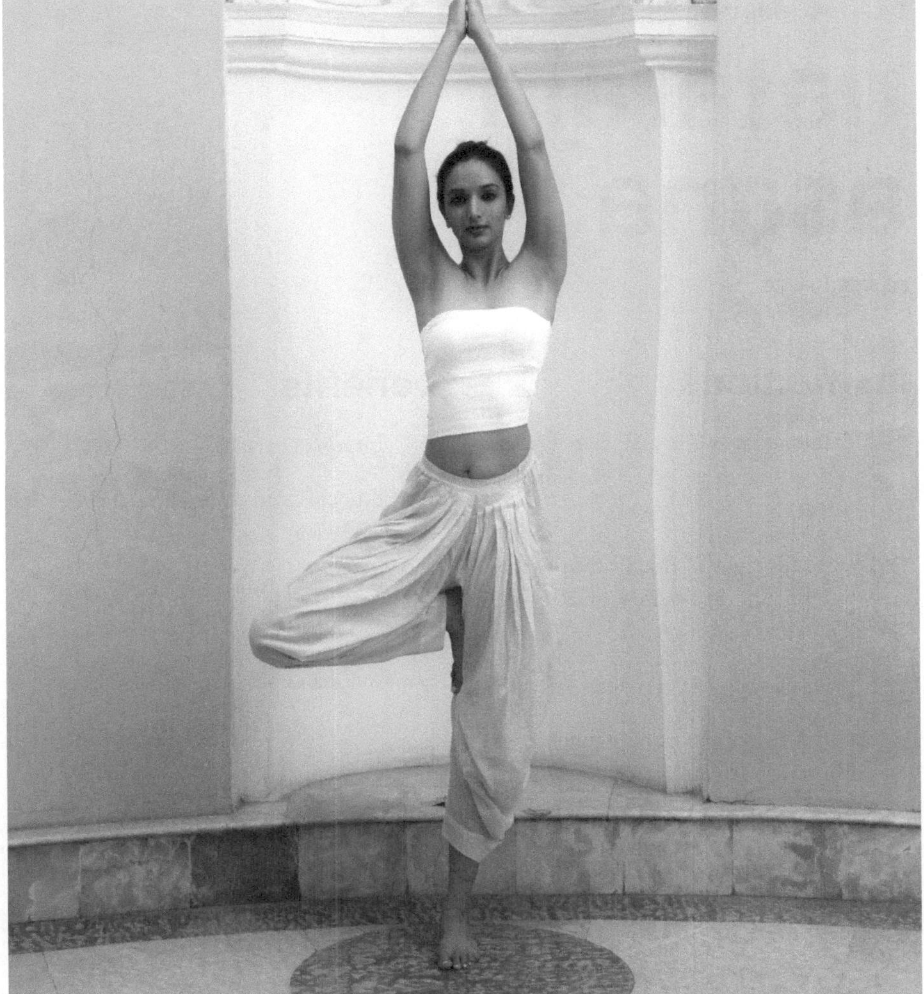

03 – TWO MINUTES

tadasana

TREE POSE

REFER TO PAGE 116

04 – TWO MINUTES

nataraja asana

DANCER POSE

instructions

1. Standing up on the mat, lean forward slightly and extend the right leg backwards
2. Bend the right knee and shifting the weight onto the left foot; grab the right foot with the right hand
3. Bring the left arm up by the ear
4. Direct the gaze towards a point in front of you to maintain balance and focus. Inhale and exhale, pulling the foot higher to stabilize the pose
5. Repeat on the other side

benefits

1. Improves balance
2. Stretches and strengthens the muscles of the leg
3. Relieves tension in the spine

contraindications: Knee injuries, spinal injuries

YOGA FACT:
This is one of yoga's most beautiful asanas. One of my favourites! Once you build your focus and get comfortable in this asana, you'll be able to feel just how graceful it is.

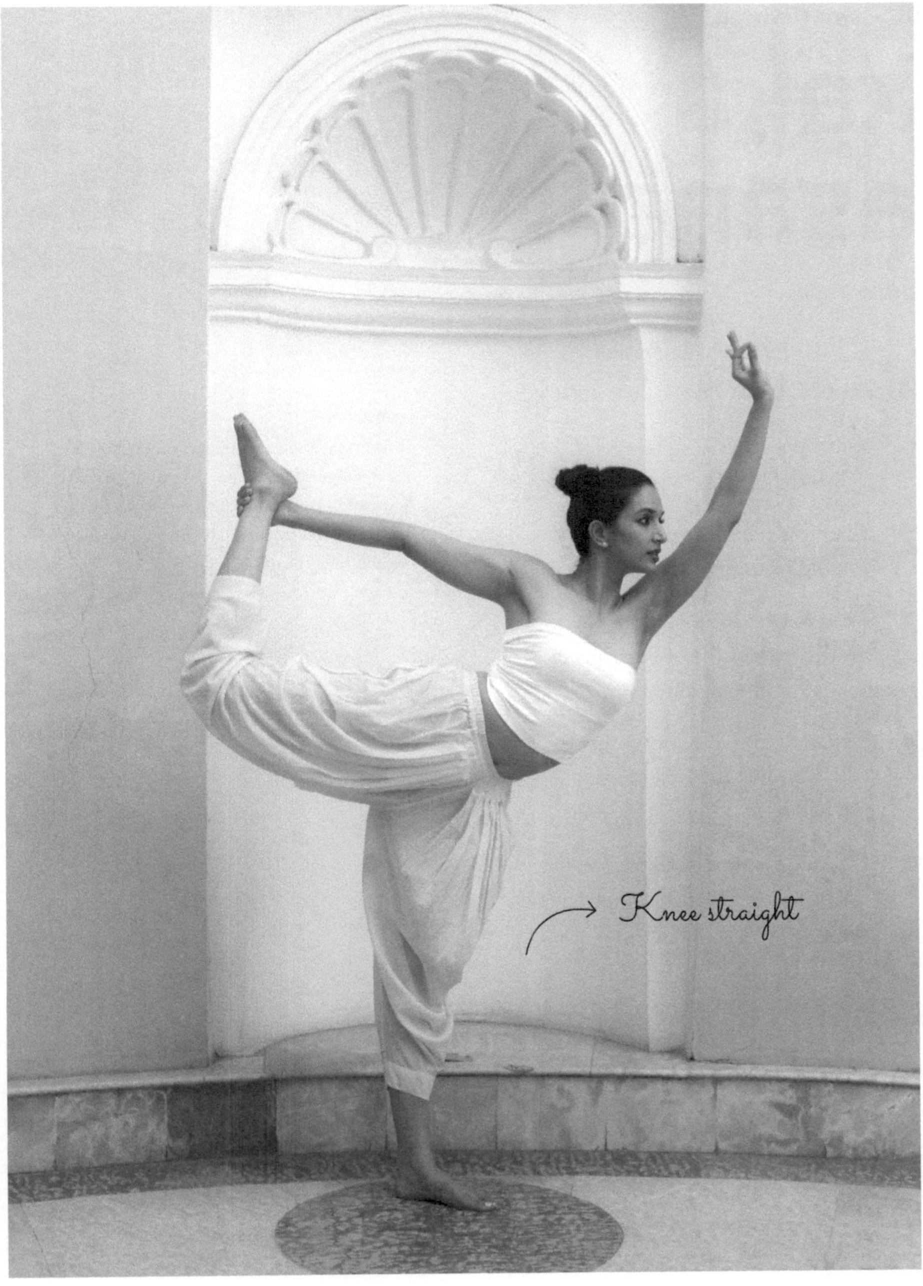
Knee straight

05 – TWO MINUTES

kaka asana

CROW POSE

instructions

1. Start in a squat with feet comfortably apart
2. Place the palms firmly on the ground in front of the feet
3. Lean forward and rest the knees on the back of the upper arms in the crook of your elbows
4. Engaging the core, slowly lift the pelvis to shift the weight into the hands
5. Lift one foot and then progressively the second to balance completely on the arms

benefits

1. Strengthens the shoulders, arms, wrists and hands
2. Strengthens abdominal muscles

contraindications: Pregnancy

YOGA TIP:
This may look like a difficult asana but it is all about gaining balance. Fix your gaze at a few feet in front of you and see how easy this becomes! You can begin by lifting just one leg up and then the other.

your notes:

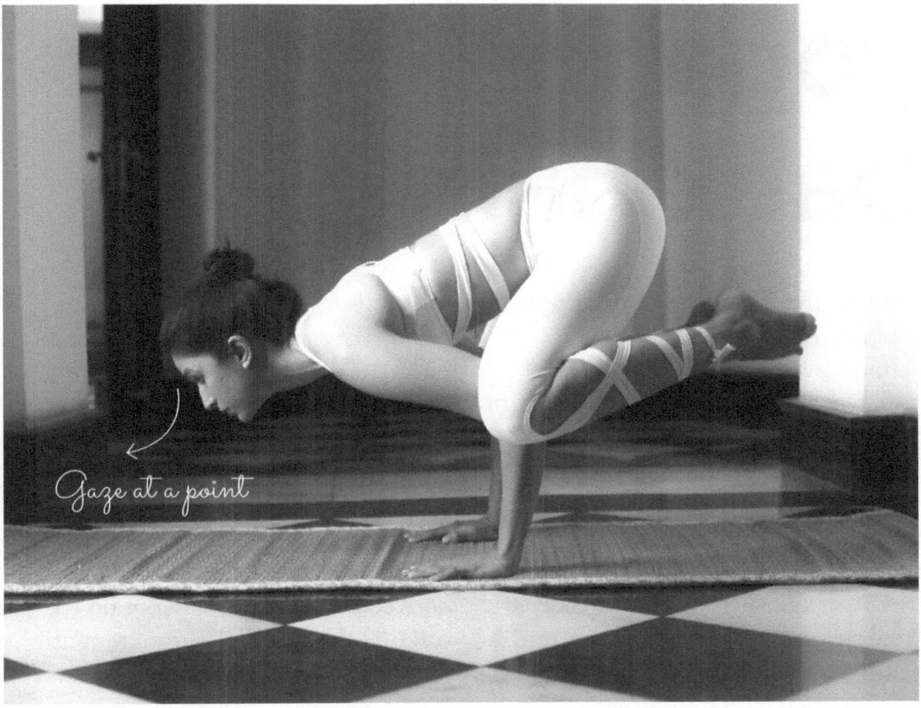

Balance is not something that you find, it is something that you create.

yoga for back pain

Perhaps the most common lifestyle problem of our time is back pain. Almost everyone that I know has suffered from back pain at some point in their lives. And it just seems to be getting worse. So many people – starting at age thirteen and going up to ninety – come to me looking for a yoga solution for this ailment. The routine below is the one I have tried, tested and perfected over ten years, for I too have suffered from terrible back pain and sometimes still do; especially during long writing stints where I put my back through extreme stress. From personal experience, I can tell you that back pain extends beyond the physical and manifests itself as fear in your minds. Everything then becomes a hazard – driving, running, walking, bending, and you go further and further down the rabbit hole till the day you decide to haul yourselves out. Yoga is known to be an amazing cure for back troubles. In fact, most physiotherapy exercises have been derived from yoga. Why not do the original then? This 10-minute routine targets each part of your back. Even if you have pain only in one part, say the neck, remember that your entire back is connected by your spine, and it is crucial to work out the whole back in its entirety to get lasting and permanent relief.

your notes:

01 – TWO MINUTES

bitalasana

CAT COW POSE

REFER TO PAGE 46

your notes:

---

02 – TWO MINUTES

salamba bhujangasana

SPHINX POSE

instructions

1. Lie face down on the stomach with arms on either side of the body
2. Placing the forearms on the floor parallel to each other push the pelvis toward the ground and raise the chest
3. Tilt the head back slightly. This helps elongate the spine and create some length in the back

benefits

1. Strengthens the spine
2. Stretches the chest and relaxes the shoulders
3. Improves blood circulation
4. Relieves stress

contraindications: Pregnancy, fractured ribs, fractured wrists

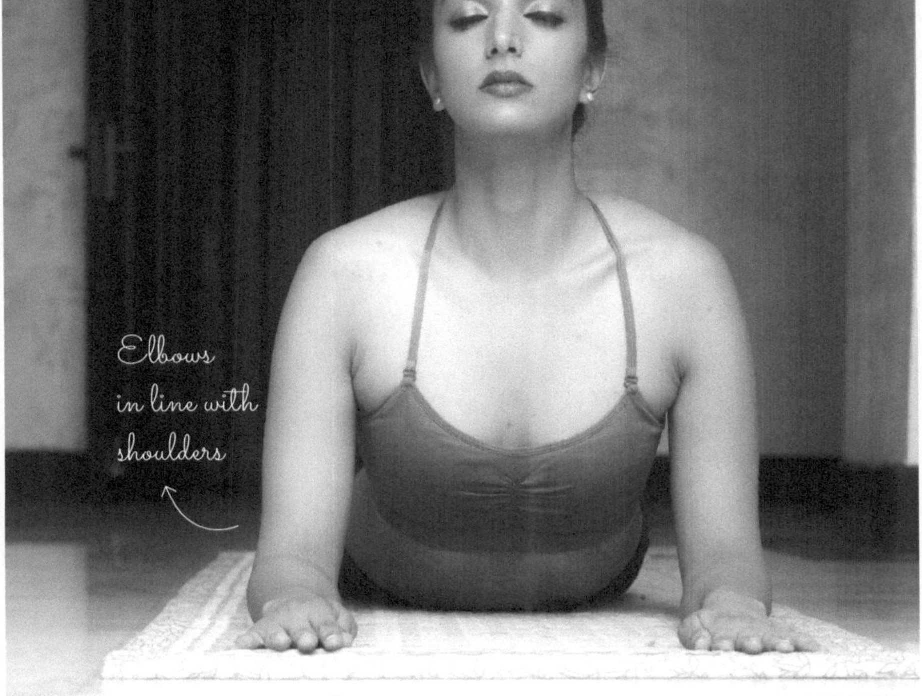
Elbows
in line with
shoulders

03 – TWO MINUTES

ardha shalabhasana

LOCUST POSE

instructions

1 Lie face down on the stomach with arms on either side of the body

2 Slide the left and right hand under the left and right hip respectively for traction

3 Inhale and lift the right leg pointing the right foot towards the ceiling as high as possible

4 Keeping the hips firmly on the ground, inhale and exhale for as long as you are comfortable

5 Exhale and lower the right leg

6 Repeat on the other side

benefits

1 Strengthens the lower back muscles

2 Relieves symptoms of indigestion, flatulence and constipation

3 Alleviates fatigue

contraindications: Headaches, spinal injuries, back injuries, neck injuries

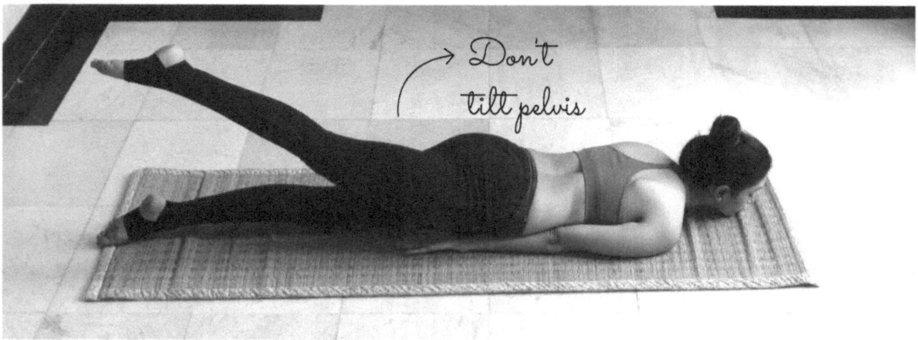

04 – TWO MINUTES

ardha matsyendra asana

LORD OF THE FISHES POSE

REFER TO PAGE 158

your notes:

05– TWO MINUTES

matsya kridasana

FLAPPING FISH POSE

REFER TO PAGE 88

As you relax in this asana, bring attention to your spine and breathe deeply. Don't underestimate this one. The simpler the asanas, the better they are for you because you can hold them longer.

your notes:

It does not matter how slowly you go as long as you do not stop.

– Confucius

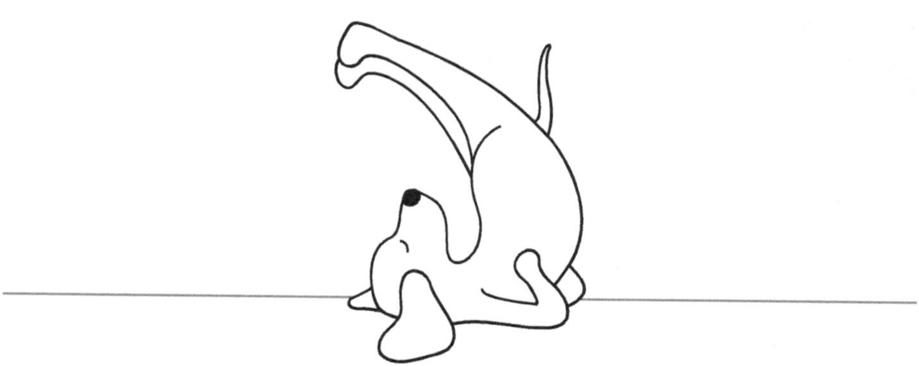

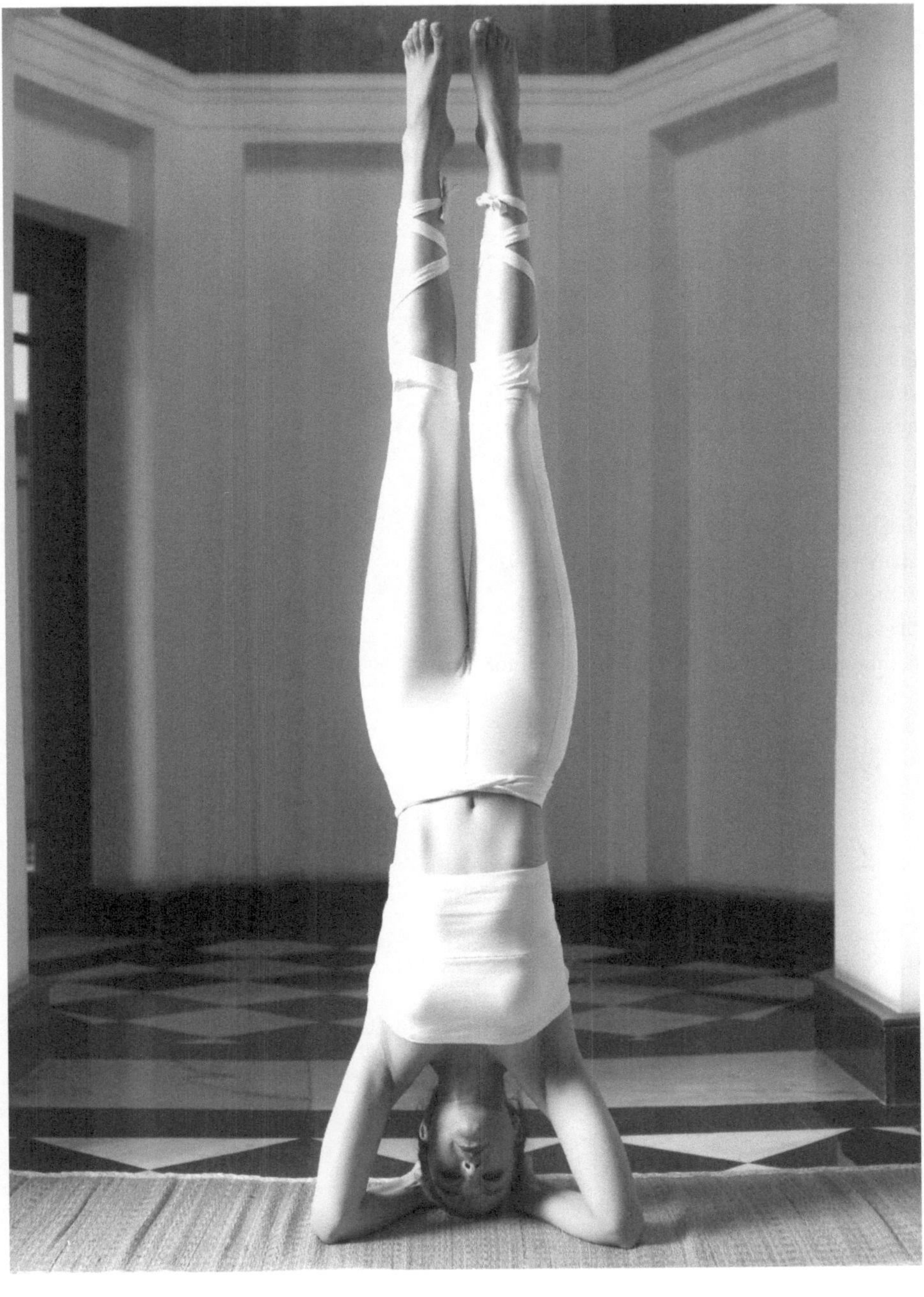

Endnote

Congratulations! You have reached the end of the 10-minute yoga solution.

While the goal of this book is to introduce you to yoga and give you short but effective solutions, the hope of this book is that you increase the time you spend practising yoga and gradually increase your practise from 10 minutes, to 20, 40 and then 60 minutes.

Yoga has changed my life. It gives me the flexibility and strength to deal with life's many twists, turns and challenges. I know, without an iota of doubt, that it can do the same for you. Thank you so much for taking out the time to read this book and for practising with me.

See you on the mat!

Namaste!
Ira

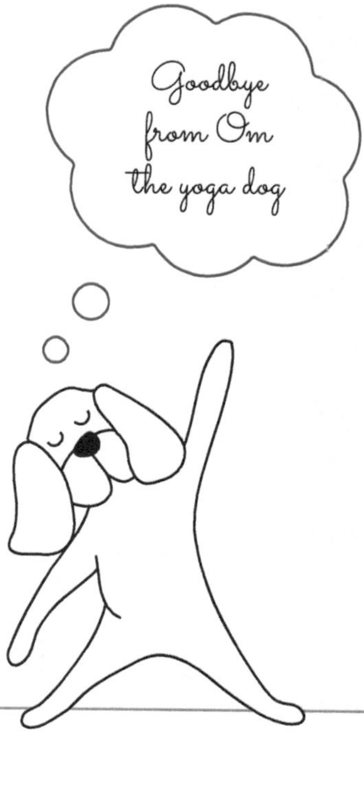

Om Tat Sat

Acknowledgements

The *10-minute Yoga Solution* is the result of a lot back-bending work. I would like to thank my parents for always encouraging me. Without support, you will fall. They are the imaginary wall behind the headstand.

A special thanks to all my yoga teachers and friends at the Sivananda Ashram, particularly Aanchal Pilani and Piyush Ghai. While yoga is a solitary journey, it always helps to have good friends along for the ride.

I would like to thank India Today Television and everyone involved in the birth of my show Yogaira, from Rahul Kanwal, Mohit Sharma, Sujay Bhattacharya and to the dedicated production and camera crew.

Thank you to the entire team at HarperCollins and Kanika Anand, my design expert. A special thanks to Ananth Padmanabhan at HarperCollins for always being a pillar of support.

AUTHOR BIO

Ira Trivedi is a bestselling author and acharya of yoga. She was part of the team that led the first international yoga day celebrations at Rajpath, which created the Guinness Book of World Records for the largest yoga class in history. She is the founder of Namami Yoga, an NGO which supports underprivileged children and the creator of Om the yoga dog. More on Ira can be found on *www.iratrivedi.in.*

Twitter @iratrivedi
IG @iratrivedi

Be happy, stay healthy, join the yogalution!

NAMAMI YOGA